Preface

Lower back pain, a broken elbow, constipation, diarrhea, and IBS all struck me during my teen years. Appendicitis, gout, and uveitis appeared in my twenties. I lived my early years in a way that led to numerous health issues. Chronic diseases typically associated with older individuals manifested in me at a young age. Even my broken elbow resulted from a mishap at age 17 while out drinking; I slipped on some algae near the docks where I lived.

As health problems piled up, I continued living as I always had, relying on pain pills as needed and occasionally taking some preemptively before a night out, just in case. I grew up in a place where going out and drinking seemed like the only option. When the sun graced London with a rare sunny day, my initial thought (sometimes still is), *'Wouldn't it be nice to be in a beer garden now?'* On Wednesday afternoons at work, my excitement to finish the day stemmed from anticipating Thursday, the start of my weekend. It was the only day I looked forward to work, as I could sneak in a few beers during lunch, and I always went out for a beer after work on Thursdays. Fridays mirrored Thursdays, but the drinking extended into the early hours. After four or five hours of sleep, I was up again for the big one – Saturday.

Saturday was the best day; no work meant I could drink all day. In the morning, my friends and I headed to the pub on an empty stomach, sometimes stopping at the pie and mash shop before returning to the pub or the working man's social club. We drank all day, extending into the evening until the early morning hours. Coming home at 6 am or 7 am was standard; sometimes, we partied through to early Sunday evening. Sundays were typically leisurely, spent in the pub after a lay-in, still usually on an empty stomach, drinking until the night's end, followed by a takeaway on the way home. On Mondays, I might attend "Monday Club" down the pub after work – a gathering for those unwilling to let go of the weekend. This was my life, emulating that of a hard-drinking middle-aged man from around 16 to 21.

It's no surprise that my health rapidly declined during this time. It wasn't the discomfort or fear of health issues that first prompted me to reconsider my lifestyle, as you'll read later. Instead, it was a brusque doctor who yelled at me over the phone, instructing me to follow his advice. This encounter led me to seek my own path forward seriously. My stubborn nature drove me on a journey to find solutions that people insisted didn't exist. Since then, I've traveled the world, meeting alternative doctors (though I dislike that term). Many were mainstream doctors who, sadly, became ill themselves or had a close family member facing illness. In desperation, they turned to therapies beyond standard medical care and, to their surprise, discovered a world they still find hard to believe. I've heard the same story repeatedly from many different doctors.

Medication can be a lifesaver, but it can also pose significant dangers. In the United States alone, annually, prescription medicine taken as prescribed is responsible for approximately 120,000 deaths. At the last check, it ranked as the 3rd to 5th leading cause of death in the United States, depending on the year— a staggering statistic. Commonly prescribed drugs for acid reflux, constipation, and other digestive issues, as well as statins and blood pressure medications, contribute significantly to these numbers. It's crucial for people to be aware that there are natural remedies that can help alleviate the reliance on prescription drugs. While I cannot make guarantees or medical claims, I

19 Natural HEALING REMEDIES That Work

From Acid Reflux To Gout,
A Guide To Using Herbs And Foods
At Home To Easily Reverse Common Diseases

ArchBrook Publishing

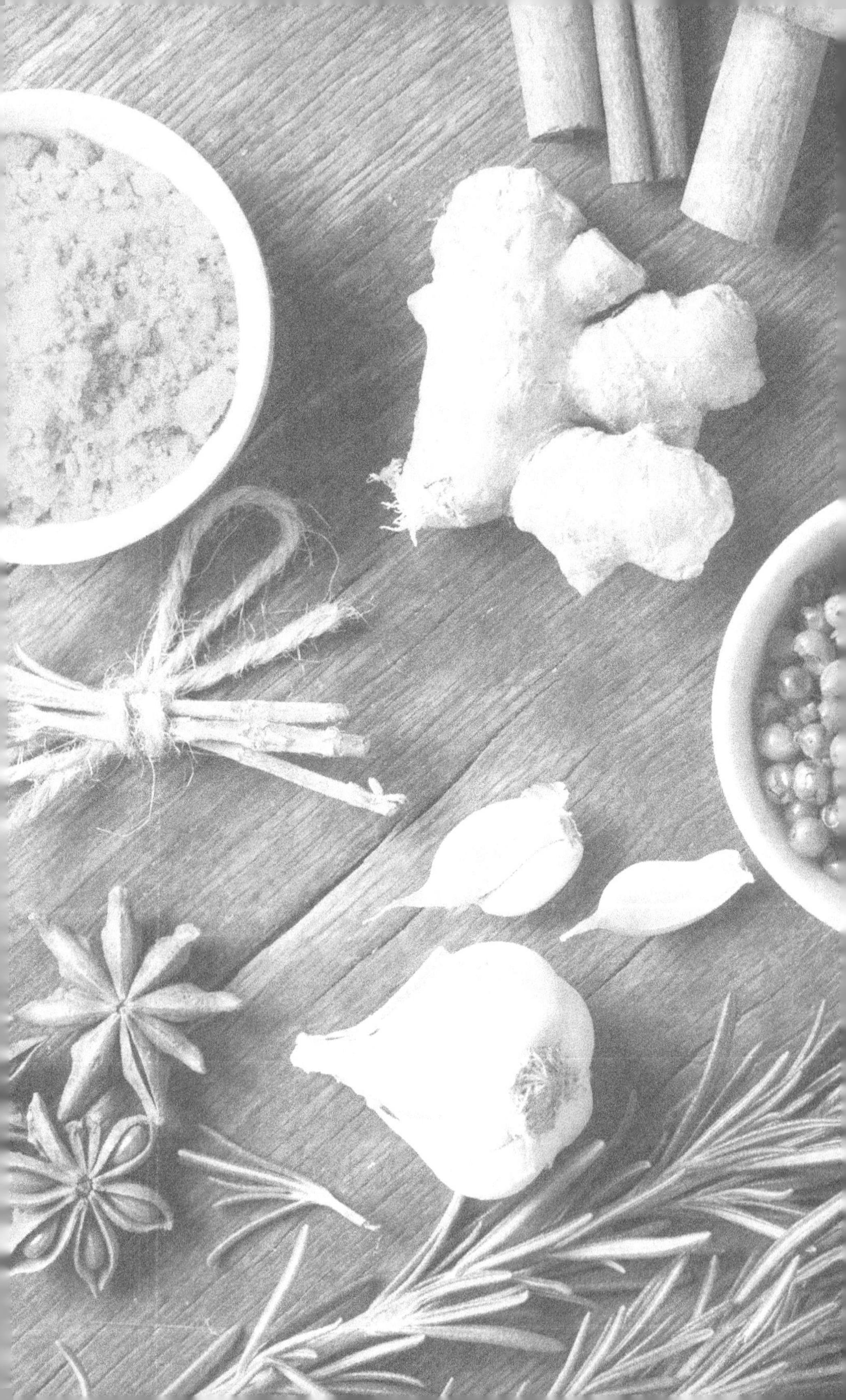

can share my observations.

This book focuses on well-established and tested natural remedies that utilize inexpensive and readily available foods and herbs. These remedies, proven to be powerful, can be affordably accessed by almost anyone and have the potential to be life-changing. I present natural solutions for common ailments prevalent in the Western world, including acid reflux, bloating, constipation, coughs, colds, flu, circulatory issues, lung problems, and the specific concern that propelled me on a quest for more information—Gout.

It's important to note that this book makes no medical claims. Instead, I encourage individuals to explore the benefits of foods and herbs traditionally known to support the body's structure and function. I advocate trying these remedies and observing their impact. While some of these 19 natural healing remedies may prove effective for you, others may not, but it's worth the attempt. Personally, I have successfully addressed my own issues, such as gout, back pain, and stomach and bowel problems, and I believe you can, too.

Disclaimer

The 19 natural healing remedies presented in this book have been personally tried and tested by numerous others, including me. Nevertheless, it's crucial to acknowledge that every individual is unique, and responses to foods and herbs, similar to medical drugs, can differ. Women that are pregnant or breastfeeding, and people taking medication, in particular, should speak to a medical practitioner before using any remedy from this book.

Please interpret this information as entertainment rather than medical advice. The author and publisher disclaim responsibility for any adverse reactions that may occur while using the information in this book. Always consult with your medical practitioner before initiating any new remedy.

Contents

Introduction

There are lots of books about natural healing remedies out there - why do we need another one?

That's what I thought to myself when I finally gave in to friends and family who, for many years, have told me that I should put all the natural healing remedies I have given them to help them overcome their health challenges into a book. All of them would be way too many! I have tried numerous natural remedies since I started on this journey.

In my quest for healing, I scoured online sources and bookshops and even visited YouTube. I discovered many "remedies" were merely generic amidst the many recommendations, echoing what others had written. While these approaches may work for some, my journey often involved experimenting with natural remedies that showed little to no noticeable effects. There seemed to be a scarcity of authentic recommendations, with few people sharing what worked for them. The 19 natural healing remedies presented in this book, however, have proven to be truly remarkable in my experience. Reflecting on my misspent youth, I now like to think that I inadvertently did the world a favor by embarking on this journey.

My teenage years were marked by severe abuse to my body—poor eating habits, excessive alcohol consumption, and chronic sleep deprivation led to the onset of degenerative diseases. Lower back pain plagued me from a young age to the extent that walking became a daunting task. A simple trip to the shops, typically a 15-minute walk, took nearly two hours. My local doctor dismissed it as growing pains. Constipation and diarrhea had been constant companions since childhood, with a doctor suggesting IBS at the age of 16.

At 17, I experienced a different kind of challenge—breaking my elbow. While not a chronic disease, the encounter provided valuable insights into the workings of doctors and hospitals. Appendicitis struck at 21, followed by a bout of gout that persisted from 23 to 30. Uveitis made its appearance at 27. In addition to these health challenges, I underwent the placement and subsequent removal of 17 mercury fillings in my teeth during my time in India. Later, I had six badly infected teeth removed in one session by a 'holistic' dentist in England. While the removal experience is vivid in my memory, it was a necessary step as teeth and root infections can surprisingly contribute to various health issues.

I have always been stubborn. I have never liked being told what to do, yet I have an open mind and an inquisitive nature. These are three qualities about me I am only now beginning to appreciate.

Rather than sit back and drift into middle age with more and more chronic health issues, I decided that I had got myself into these health issues, so I would get myself out! I chose to study and obtain qualifications in herbalism, nutrition, nutritional therapy, anatomy, physiology, and sports electrotherapy, to name just a few. The idea was to learn what works and use it on myself, friends, and family (if I could convince them). I soon learned that, although the basic learning was good, I never saw stunning results. And I knew stunning results were possible. One day, I made what seemed to me to be a massive realization. I had a lightbulb moment. <u>I realized you **never** hear of miraculous health recoveries in ANY official mainstream therapy method. No one reverses chronic disease.</u> Emergency medicine, people being fixed after car accidents, and the like, yes, it is amazing. Yet, no one went to their rheumatologist and got 100% better. You just get given drugs to help ease the pain while the horrible degeneration continues. And for some reason, that is the accepted way.

But not for me. I had heard of miracles. I knew people who had reversed serious diseases with nutritional approaches and devices such as Cold Lasers, Pulsed Electromagnetic Therapy, Hydrogen Inhalation Therapy, and many others. But these things were not 'mainstream.' Why?

I started working with people briefly and loved to help them, so much so that it showed just how bad a businessman I am. I gave away my time, products I'd sourced, and therapy sessions for free. I quickly discovered that giving anything away for free isn't a good thing. People don't respect free. People don't value free, even when they get AMAZING results. I think people don't trust anything free to work. I can only assume the thought process goes something like this: "If this works, if it is so good, why is it free? Also, why can't I get this from my doctor? If it works, they will use it!" That could not be further from the truth. This frustrated me about working with people. Don't get me wrong, I can be the same. I have spent a fortune, literally traveling around the world, seeing doctors to help me with my issues using their 'alternative' methods. I have spent tens of thousands of pounds on equipment and not used it as instructed. Humans are complex animals!

Discovering the 19 natural healing remedies I share in this book resulted from what I like to call unstructured learning. This involved delving into books, ranging from very old to contemporary, scouring online sources from Google to Pubmed. One remarkable figure I encountered in my research was Tony Pantalleresco, a nutty-professor genius from

Canada. Tony employs herbs and foods in a unique manner, thinking outside the conventional boundaries and engaging in what he termed 15 years ago as "food alchemy." I stumbled upon Tony's insights through YouTube, made contact, delved into his books and research material, and was genuinely mind-blown by his approach.

My exploration also led me to the wisdom of herbalists from bygone years, such as Susan Weed and David Winston. While Neal's Yard has published some excellent books, none quite matched the depth of Tony's information. I've honed in on what works through extensive trial and error, testing hundreds of natural remedies on myself and others. Tony's influence was pivotal, and I express my gratitude to him for inspiring some of the 19 natural healing remedies in this book.

While I hold great respect for the mainstream medical system, acknowledging its role in saving lives, including mine and my brother's, during a severe bout of appendicitis, I've also witnessed its limitations, particularly in addressing chronic diseases. In my view, modern medicine should play a role specifically in emergency medicine, dealing with accidents, acute emergencies, and necessary joint replacements—areas where it undeniably excels. However, when it comes to chronic diseases, my perspective is different. To my knowledge, mainstream medicine hasn't eradicated a single chronic disease. For instance, in my early twenties, I was advised to take gout tablets daily for the rest of my life. Dissatisfied with this solution, I questioned the doctor about the necessity and the high dosage. It struck me as odd that my sister's husband, who had severe gout in his knees, was prescribed less than half the dose of Allopurinol that I received.

The doctor's response, a shouted command to "Just take what you have been given," still resonates with me to this day. Working on a construction project, building the 2012 Olympic Stadium in London, I found myself walking up and down the office corridor, engaged in a heated exchange with the doctor over the phone. His lack of explanation and refusal to discuss the prescribed pill infuriated me. I don't appreciate being shouted at, and the absence of a meaningful conversation only fueled my frustration. Aware that committing to taking this particular drug was a lifelong decision, I knew that every medication comes with side effects and depletes certain nutrients in the human body—an aspect doctors should inform patients about. This information can be found on various websites, and anyone taking a medication long term should consider researching them, as nutrient deficiencies can lead to health issues down the road.

I can be stubborn, and the doctor's approach didn't sit well with me, and it seemed he lacked a clear understanding. Consequently, I opted not to take the pill. This decision propelled me on a mission to find a solution for my gout on my own and find a cure. And I did. This experience opened my eyes and mind to the realization that there are alternative ways to address health issues and that not all doctors possess the necessary insights. The remedy that ultimately eradicated my gout, which is featured as number 19 in the Remedy section of this book, became the catalyst for my transformative journey.

It dawned on me that a concoction of pineapple, aloe vera juice, and certain spices could be more effective than a medical drug. Unlike pharmaceuticals, my special anti-gout juice yielded positive side effects such as improved circulation, reduced inflammation, and overall hydration, among other benefits.

The positive outcomes I experienced fueled my determination to explore and share more natural healing remedies, and the feedback I received was overwhelmingly positive. The joy of imparting information that positively transforms someone's life is unparalleled. I firmly believe that the health issues afflicting millions daily can be reversed. I am convinced your local grocery store can provide foods and herbs to alleviate conditions ranging from constipation, acid reflux, gout, coughs, and colds to diabetes, gas bloating, and arthritis.

Life will inevitably present health challenges. I urge you to explore your spice rack and food cupboard for potential solutions. You will be amazed at what you find.

Section 1

We Used To Use Herbs, But Now We Have REAL Medicine. Right?

It is a common misconception that humans have evolved using herbs and plants as medicine for over millennia. But then, we found a much better, more advanced healing method in modern medicine and pharmaceutical drugs.

Don't get me wrong, modern medicine in all its forms can be amazing. Infections that were once a life-or-death situation can now be overcome with just five days of taking a pill or two daily while getting on with your life. Emergency heart surgery and other surgeries, such as joint replacement surgeries, are absolutely mind-boggling, and we are lucky to have such emergency procedures. That said, I believe modern medicine is suited as 'Emergency Medicine.' Most 'chronic' diseases are a side effect of modern living and eating, which no drug can reverse. Antibiotics kill bacteria, steroids significantly reduce inflammation, and painkillers can take away annoying daily aches, pains, and even high-level pain caused by trauma. This is all great! But what are the consequences?

As I'm writing this, the United States spends the most on modern medicine, so you may think they have amazing health outcomes when going to the hospital. But they don't, and it's easy to see why.

Antibiotics kill bacteria to give our body's immune system a chance to get together and overcome infections. This is amazing, but it is common knowledge that doctors have overused antibiotics, and this, unfortunately, has led to antibiotic-resistant infections. Oh dear. At the same time, antibiotics also kill the bacteria in our bodies that do good things for us, like keeping yeast in check, those that create nutrients for us, and much more. That is why thrush is common among women that use antibiotics. "Good bacteria," as they are known, also interact with our immune and hormone systems. This means that when we kill them, things go wrong. This science is still in its infancy but is fascinating and very important.

Prescription painkillers kill and seriously injure many thousands in the United States alone every year. In fact, doctors' mistakes added to "deaths from prescription drugs," which we could group together as a 'modern medicine' category, are THE leading killer in the United States, beating cancer and heart disease. Now, that is something to think about.

This is not an anti-Modern Medicine rant, by the way. Not at all. As I have said already, emergency medicine has saved my life. But something has to be wrong when the leading cause of death in a country that spends more money on health care than the top 10 Countries behind them spend combined is the very thing that all that money is spent on. This is crazy to me, and the people of the United States and we in the United Kingdom deserve better.

While significant profits are generated within our current medical system, where drug companies earn billions of dollars annually by providing medications that merely suppress symptoms of diseases without offering cures, can you imagine a scenario where we are presented with a cure for any chronic disease?"

The United States and the United Kingdom should be right up there in world health and longevity stats. But as of today, 06/11/2023, the website, www.worldometers.info, shows the following information.

Average Life Expectancy Age Top 100 Countries:
UK ranks at Number 30
US ranks at Number 47

Despite all that money spent on what is described as 'health care' in the United States, FORTY-SIX countries have a population that lives longer on average. This is a worrying statistic.

The statistics for live births and first-year survival of babies are just as bad. Last I read, the United States ranked number 41 on the list. How on earth does that happen when you spend more than the rest of the world by multiple billions of dollars? Something to really think about is that babies from FORTY countries have more chances to be born and survive their first year than those in the first-world country of the United States of America. To me, this is shocking. Truly shocking.

Doctors do not generally like to treat vast amounts of patients in very little time. But they must. We are allocated 7 minutes with our local GP. Also, doctors' education is now largely infiltrated by pharmaceutical companies, which has brought them to a strange place where they match symptoms to medication. Gone are the days when doctors had the time to get to know their patients, their history, and their daily lives. Doctors used to touch, closely examine, and even smell patients to properly diagnose them. Right now, we are fast approaching a time when AI bots, not a doctor, will be our first port of call to check symptoms. This technology is being worked on now, and I find this "progress" very scary.

Doctors, just like the rest of us, don't know what they don't know. It's not always their fault. The medical system has simply failed.

Nevertheless, I do hold doctors accountable, such as the one who advised me to take medication daily for the rest of my life. I also blame the doctors who recommended my four-year-old son use an inhaler pump daily for the rest of his life despite him not needing one. Furthermore, the doctors who suggested my wife give our 10-month-old daughter both antihistamine and a broad-spectrum antibiotic 'just in case' when her hand became swollen without proper diagnosis—I hold them responsible. Why? Because their decisions stemmed from laziness and a desire to cover their own backs, and the potential negative impacts of these prescriptions could have affected our health for a lifetime. Regrettably, our experiences are not isolated incidents within my family. I can sadly recount many instances of subpar medical practices.

However, this isn't an exercise in doctor-bashing. Rather, it's crucial to acknowledge that doctors and modern medicine don't possess all the answers. Just because they might be unaware of the incredible natural remedies available doesn't negate their existence. Undoubtedly, there are remarkable natural solutions that could prove beneficial for you or your loved ones.

In the current landscape, having access to easily-created natural remedies at home may be more important than ever.

Why Are Natural Remedies Important?

Many people believe that natural remedies are for hippies who hug trees and don't want to get along with the times. There's also the mistaken belief that in our current civilized state, with advanced technology and scientific breakthroughs enabling drug creation, we no longer require the use of herbs. This is completely untrue.

It is now widely recognised that most modern chronic diseases are caused by environmental factors. This means the things you eat and drink, the nutrients you don't get, the toxic substances you do get, the sleep or lack of sleep, etc., could be the cause of the disease. This means drugs alone will never be able to reverse a disease. Diseases are not caused by a lack of painkillers or lack of other drugs. Diseases are caused by a lack of essential nutrients, lack of sleep, too much stress, a lowered immune system, environmental toxins, etc. To fix the root cause of any disease, you need to get the essential nutrients into your body and system, sleep properly, de-stress and use nature's bounty of complex compounds found in foods and herbs. These are the same foods and herbs we have evolved with over time, and they will help you get back to health.

The pharmaceutical industry is becoming extortionately expensive. This is extremely worrying in countries like the United States and the United Kingdom. It is even now a concern for Asian countries such as India, where people need to have insurance or pay for drugs out of their own pocket. It would be great if people could take a preventative approach to health, but many of us don't.

The good news is that the human body is AMAZING. It is self-healing (you didn't think doctors healed you, did you?) and fantastically adapting. It has the ability to compensate for times when we don't do the things we should do. When we stop doing the things that cause issues and begin to give the human body natural remedies, the human body can heal. Combining simple everyday foods and herbs can achieve wonderful results, from constipation to acid reflux to gout and viral infections.

This may sound like an over-exaggeration to some people. I mean, what can a herb do that a drug can't?

Let's take ginger.

Over 400 complex compounds are found in ginger. We know what some of them do; that's why a Canadian pharmaceutical company isolated gingerols from ginger, chemically altered the molecule and tried to patent it as an anti-cancer drug many years ago. If you look on official medical research sites such as Pubmed, you will see them list the anti-cancer effects of ginger.

In fact, ginger's cousins, turmeric and, even more impressive, galangal, also have many scientific papers showing their ability to fight various forms of cancer. The issue is pharmaceutical companies cannot patent ginger or even a specific chemical in ginger. They would have to alter the molecule so they can patent it. That could mean it could also cause an altered outcome in the human body.

Traditional herbalists will tell you that the whole plant is often much superior to an extract of one chemical of a plant. So, what do you think happens when you take whole ginger and juice it with turmeric, pineapple, and celery? We have profiles of the foods we use in the 19 natural healing remedies later in this book but do a little google search on what plant compounds are in each of those four foods. Ask Google or Chat GPT for the health benefits of each food item or even deep dive into the nutrients contained within them. You will be surprised. Pharmaceutical companies would love to have a drug that can do what ginger can do.

And the best thing is you have direct access to foods and herbs, and you can utilize them TODAY!

The 19 natural healing remedies I have for you are amazing, tried and tested. Although there are some things we need to be careful with, mostly, the side effects you may experience are improved health and a longer, happier, more energized life.

Do They Really Work?

In a nutshell, YES. That said, I cannot make any guarantees.

People are skeptical about "natural remedies," probably because the word "remedy" is old-fashioned. Today, doctors don't talk about natural remedies (or cures, unfortunately) but only about drugs and disease management.

When someone experiences pain, they are often offered pain management medications with the assurance, 'We can help manage your symptoms.' Rarely does one hear a doctor declare an intention to cure the ailment, except in cases of infections where antibiotics are still effective. It's striking how modern science has made significant strides in various fields, from car mechanics to computing technologies. Yet, medical science, in many aspects, appears to have lagged behind. While surgical techniques have advanced, the outright cure or prevention of chronic diseases remains elusive.

Conditions such as heart disease, cancer, diabetes, and even autism seem to be not just on the rise in proportion to the population but growing exponentially. Twenty years ago, autism was a rare 1 in 10,000 occurrence. But now it affects 1 in 100 people—a concerning trend that doesn't reflect progress. Each year, new diseases are discovered or at least 'named,' with a growing emphasis on relying on pills for every ailment and less on addressing factors like diet, nutrition, and lifestyle. It seems evident to me that we need to shift our focus in that direction.

Luckily, the 'health industry' is rapidly growing in response to more and more people getting sick. More people are beginning to stop listening to the mainstream narrative. They are starting out on their personal journey, looking for a different way, just as I did many years ago. Certain diets have become popular, fads they may be, but people are finding that their health issues go away or are markedly improved when they go vegan or try paleo, keto, or carnivore. Vegan and carnivore are two completely opposite diets, so how and why are people reversing autoimmune diseases with both? People with cancer are turning to vegan-like diets. Juicing lots of fruit and vegetables as per Gerson Therapy and the like. Others have found that a keto diet has helped. The one thing I have noticed is that all these diets tend to cut out processed foods and sugar. People are now health conscious and usually eat whole foods, start exercising, and even turn to meditation. Lo and behold, their disease goes away with diet and lifestyle changes.

Foods and herbs are complex, containing many nutrients and plant chemicals that the human body needs. Make no mistake, the 19 natural healing remedies in this book work, and that's one reason you need to be cautious when using them. These foods and herbs are potent.

Mostly, any negative side effects might be that it tastes bad or possibly causes an upset stomach. However, these 19 natural healing remedies can increase the uptake of drugs, so please take caution when using them. <u>All natural remedies should be taken two hours away from drug medication.</u>

Section 2

The Food, Herbs and Products we use

When thinking about what natural healing remedies would be worthy of writing down in a book, I needed criteria to work with. This is what I came up with

- Firstly, the 19 natural healing remedies had to work. I have used them and had multiple people give solid feedback that they have worked for them, too.
- They must be multifunctional. Unlike taking a specific drug for a specific 'thing',natural food and herbal remedies should have wide-reaching benefits. That means the 19 natural healing remedies have many more uses than just 19.
- Relatively cheap ingredients and readily available in most countries.
- The 19 natural healing remedies would have crossover ingredients. I didn't want to have 19 different remedies that needed 187 ingredients to create them.
- The 19 natural healing remedies had to be relatively easy and quick to make. No making something and having to wait six months to use it.
- The 19 natural healing remedies can be made by anyone. Although you must respect the end product, this isn't a lab-grade experiment whereby if you get a measurement wrong, it will be wasted. Just make sure you read the cautions.
- Safe! As per the disclaimer, there are some precautions, especially if you are pregnant or breastfeeding, don't use these for obvious

reasons, but in general, we are not creating anything unsafe.

- Finally, I had to stick to the 19 natural healing remedies. I have offered a couple of supplements to use. But for the most part, I have decided to leave vitamin and mineral supplements and other health supplements out of these 19 natural healing remedies.

Part of the criteria was going to be that they taste good. There is an old saying, "It doesn't matter how good a remedy is if no one will take it." This is a valid point. However, I realized that I would either leave out the best, most effective, health-enhancing remedies or add a ton more ingredients to try and make them taste better. So, the 19 natural healing remedies are what they are. Use them, feel their benefits, and then play with the recipes to find what works for you with respect to taste and effectiveness.

Profiles

Below is a brief profile of each food, herb or product used in the 19 natural healing remedies. It is certainly not a comprehensive list of chemical constituents and biological actions. The profiles below are a brief summary that will hopefully get you thinking and playing with the items here when you have an issue.

See what you can create with what you have in your home at the first sign of a scratchy throat coming on or after a large dinner when you feel bloated and have discomfort when you never usually do. You will definitely be able to go to the 19 natural healing remedies. But you can also look through these profiles and put something together. Remember, play with it, and if you tweak things, make them better, or find something new, please share it with me at 19remediesthatwork@gmail.com

NOTE: Please use organic where you can.

Aloe Vera

Properties & Health Benefits:

- Help treat skin conditions and improve skin appearance.
- Benefit pre-diabetes treatment.
- Helps with digestion.
- May improve dental and oral health.
- Contains antioxidants.
- Moisturizes Hair and Scalp.
- Anti-Inflammatory properties
- Detoxification.
- Treats Constipation

Aloe vera is a versatile and powerful plant with a wide range of benefits for your health and well-being. Whether you're looking to improve your skin, boost your immune system, aid digestion, or address various health concerns, aloe vera is a valuable addition to your wellness routine.

Where To Buy: Aloe vera products can be found in various forms, such as gel, creams, and supplements, at health food stores, pharmacies, and online retailers. You can also grow your Aloe Vera plant at home for a fresh supply of its gel.

Cautions: Aloe latex should not be taken in high doses because it may cause adverse side effects, such as stomach pain and cramps. Long-term use of large amounts of aloe latex might also cause diarrhea, kidney problems, blood in the urine, low potassium, muscle weakness, weight loss and heart issues. Don't take aloe vera, either gel or latex, if you're pregnant or breastfeeding.

Tips: For topical applications, extract the gel from fresh aloe vera leaves for the best results. When using aloe vera for internal purposes, choose high-quality, pure aloe vera products to ensure its effectiveness and safety.

Apple Cider Vinegar

Properties & Claimed Health Benefits:

- Aids digestion
- Reduces bloating
- Can help control acid reflux
- Supports weight loss (curbs appetite)
- Helps control blood sugar
- May help lower cholesterol levels
- Treats acne and improves skin health
- Alkalizing effect on the body
- Helps fight infections
- Supports the detoxification process in the body
- Enhances hair shine and cleans the scalp

Where To Buy: You can find apple cider vinegar in most grocery and health food stores.

Cautions: Apple cider vinegar appears safe when diluted if you don't take excessive amounts of it. Avoid undiluted vinegar in dental care and skin care. Moderation is the key.

Tips: The best way to incorporate apple cider vinegar into your diet is to use it in cooking. It's a simple addition to foods like salad dressings, homemade herbal vinegar, or simply a glass of warm water.

Bicarbonate Of Soda

Properties & Claimed Health Benefits:

- Helps treat heartburn
- Soothes canker sores

- As a high alkaline, it can help relieve acid reflux
- Improve exercise performance
- Relieve itchy skin and sunburns
- May slow the progression of chronic kidney disease
- May improve certain cancer treatments
- Oral hygiene routine
- Teeth whitener
- Used for treatment of urinary tract infections
- Pesticide remover for fruits and vegetables

Baking soda is a versatile ingredient whose uses extend beyond cooking. Bicarbonate of soda has some amazing health benefits, and whole books have been written about it. Check out Dr Mark Sircus' book for a deep dive and be ready to be amazed. Examples of its benefits are helping to alleviate heartburn, boost exercise performance, and even whiten your teeth. Dr Jerry Tennant, an amazing world-famous ophthalmologist from Texas, now an integrative doctor and researcher, made the statement, "Taking ¼ teaspoon of Bicarbonate of soda in a glass of warm water every morning might be the most important thing you can do to improve your health."

Where To Buy: Bicarbonate of soda is readily available in most grocery stores, supermarkets, and pharmacies. Look for aluminum-free.

Cautions: It's essential to use bicarbonate of soda in moderation when ingested, as excessive consumption can disrupt the body's acid-base balance. Excessive use as a toothpaste may erode tooth enamel.

Tips: There are over-the-counter and prescription tablets for people who don't like the taste of baking soda. Most of them dissolve easily in water. See the instructions on the box for the recommended dosage.

Blueberries (Vaccinium corymbosum)

Properties & Health Benefits:

- Rich in antioxidants
- Can reduce DNA damage
- Help fight urinary tract infections
- Potentially help manage blood sugar (leaves)
- Potentially reduces blood pressure
- Help manage cholesterol
- Help prevent heart disease
- Help maintain brain function and improve memory
- Anthocyanins within them may have anti-diabetes effects

Blueberries are a nutritious berry and have therapeutic effects. The leaves of the blueberry bush are also used in herbalism to help treat high blood sugar levels that lead to diabetes. Often labeled a "superfood," blueberries are low in calories and taste great. Like their cousin, the bilberry, blueberries have been used for capillary health and to support healthy vision.

Where To Buy: Blueberries are widely available in most grocery stores, supermarkets, and even local farmers' markets. You can find them in the fresh produce section or the frozen fruit aisle, allowing you to enjoy their benefits year-round. Always try to get organic, or better still, grow your own!

Cautions: Blueberries are a common food and generally safe to consume.

Tips: Blueberries can be consumed in various ways, including fresh, frozen, in smoothies, or even consumed as a tincture or tea.

Brandy

Properties & Claimed Health Benefits:

- Acts as antioxidant
- May have anti-ageing properties
- Improves circulation
- Has a warming effect
- Relieve coughs and sore throats

Promoting a strong spirit as a health product is hard, but brandy, mixed with good raw local honey, has been used for a long time for coughs and colds. Modern research has shown that brandy has antioxidant and positive effects on platelet aggregation.

Where To Buy: You can purchase brandy at liquor stores, wine shops, or online retailers. It's available in various styles and brands.

Cautions: We only use very small amounts of brandy in remedies. If you have problems with alcohol, you can often use aloe vera juice instead.

Tips: I like Brandy over Vodka for Tinctures as it has added antioxidant effects of its own.

Burdock (Arctium minus)

Properties & Claimed Health Benefits:

- Used to treat skin issues
- Boosts the immune system
- Helps Balance blood sugar levels
- Supports gastrointestinal health
- Removes toxins from the blood
- Supports liver health
- Used in famous herbal cancer formulas
- Reduce Chronic Inflammation
- Diuretic

Burdock root is eaten as a vegetable in Northern Asia and Europe. Burdock root has been used for centuries in herbal medicine to treat a variety of different conditions. Traditionally, it's been mostly used as a diuretic and a digestive aid. Now, researchers have discovered numerous potential uses and health benefits for burdock root, and it has been shown to help skin issues and improve liver health.

Where To Buy: Burdock root can be found in health food stores, herbal shops, or online retailers that sell herbs and herbal products.

Cautions: Burdock's diuretic nature may worsen dehydration, especially when taken with other diuretics. Allergic reactions may occur if you are sensitive to chrysanthemums or daisies. Pregnant women or those trying to conceive should avoid Burdock root and its supplements.

Tips: Use burdock with dandelion as a pre-meal drink. It is a great digestive aid that will also help keep the blood clean.

Butter

Properties & Claimed Health Benefits:

- Rich in healthy fats
- Source of fat-soluble vitamins
- Promotes brain health
- Enhances taste and flavor
- Supports bone health
- Aids in nutrient absorption
- Suitable for low-heat cooking

Contains Conjugated Linoleic Acid (CLA), which is linked to impressive health benefits

Butter is a versatile and delicious addition to your diet; some call it a true superfood. Butter contains Vitamin A, D, E, and K2 in forms highly usable by the human body. The fats in butter build strong cell membranes and provide the raw materials to nourish the brain and the central nervous system. Adding butter to vegetables improves mineral absorption.

Where To Buy: Butter is readily available at most grocery stores and supermarkets. However, it is best to purchase from a local organic farmer that lets cows roam and eat grass. If you can get this butter, purchase it in bulk in spring. This is when butter has high amounts of vitamin K2, which is hard to get in most diets but has amazing health benefits.

Cautions: Although butter has benefits, consuming too much in one go (such as adding two tablespoons to coffee in the morning) may lead to loose bowels!

Tips: When using butter, opt for high-quality, grass-fed butter whenever possible, as it tends to have a better nutrient profile. Experiment with using butter in cooking at a low temperature or simply add to cooked vegetables.

Cayenne Pepper

Properties & Claimed Health Benefits:

- May help during a heart attack
- Boost metabolism
- Can help lower blood pressure
- Helps improve digestive health
- Improves blood circulation
- Can help with pain reduction
- Helps ease joint pain
- Clears congestion
- Protective effect on the heart
- Can help stop bleeding if used internally and topically

Cayenne Pepper has whole books written about it. A favourite of legendary herbalist Dr John Christopher, Cayenne pepper is a hot herb that improves blood flow, gets things moving in general, and can often be added to herbal tincture mixes as it is thought to help distribute other herbs around the body.

Where To Buy: You can find cayenne pepper at most grocery stores, supermarkets, or spice shops. It's available in powdered, flake, or dried form.

Cautions: Some people may be allergic to cayenne; others may have a low tolerance to using it as it is a spicy hot herb. Do not get in your eyes. If you have gastrointestinal conditions, consult your medical practitioner before using cayenne.

Tips: Cayenne pepper is a powerful spice; start with small doses, ⅛ of a teaspoon, and increase slowly.

Chamomile flowers (Chamaemelum nobile)
Properties & Claimed Health Benefits:

- Promotes digestive health
- Helps to relieve cold symptoms
- Reduces inflammation
- May help to relieve menstrual symptoms
- Can help in mild skin conditions
- Helps to maintain diabetes and blood sugar
- Improve heart health
- Boosts immune health

There are two main types of chamomiles: Roman and German. German chamomile is considered more effective for inflammatory skin issues. In contrast, Roman Chamomile is deemed superior for bowel issues, but both can be used interchangeably. Chamomile tea is a popular herb used in sleep and digestive tea formulas. Chamomile is an herb from the daisy-like flowers of the Asteraceae plant family. It has been consumed for centuries as a natural remedy for various health conditions.

Where To Buy: You can find chamomile flowers in various forms, including dried loose flowers for tea, as well as in pre-packaged tea bags, at most health food stores and online retailers.

Cautions: Although a few people may be allergic to chamomile, it is safe for most people to drink. Negative side effects are extremely rare.

Tips: Chamomile can be used in skincare routines by infusing it into oils or using chamomile-based products.

Chicken Broth

Properties & Claimed Health Benefits:

- Known as a long-standing anti-cold and flu supporter
- Contains immune-boosting amino acids.
- Abundant in essential vitamins and minerals.
- Easily digestible and soothing for the stomach.
- Provides hydration and essential nutrients.
- Rich in collagen, aiding joint health.
- Supports recovery from illnesses and surgeries.
- May enhance skin elasticity.
- Contains amino acids with potential anti-inflammatory effects.

Broth is made by simmering the bones and connective tissue of chicken. This forms a stock for making soups, sauces, and gravies. Rich in nutrients like collagen, gelatin, and glycine, chicken bone broth is friendly to the joints and provides a host of amino acids. Research has discovered that chicken broth contains a protein that directly improves Immune T and B cells.

Where To Buy: Buy chicken carcasses from a local organic farm (cheap) or use the bones of the chicken you eat. I find making it is the best and cheapest way to consume chicken broth.

Cautions: Commercial chicken broths may have a high sodium content, so individuals on a low-sodium diet should be cautious when using them. Also, individuals with poultry allergies should avoid chicken broth.

Tips: Get bones from your local butcher or farmers market to make your broth. Just 1 cup a day provides good health benefits. Consider combining it with garlic, ginger, and other herbs to boost health benefits.

Cinnamon (Cinnamomum verum)

Properties & Claimed Health Benefits:

- As a tea, it helps digestion
- Loaded with antioxidants
- Fights inflammation and infections
- Can help balance blood sugar levels
- May protect against heart disease
- Could improve sensitivity to insulin
- Balances blood sugar levels
- May have beneficial effects on neurodegenerative diseases
- May protect against cancer
- Prevent bacterial and fungal infections
- Has anti-viral properties

Cinnamon is a spice prized for its medicinal properties for thousands of years. It is a versatile spice with a wide range of health benefits. You can incorporate it into your daily routine in various ways, such as adding it to your meals, drinking it as tea, or even using it in tinctures.

Where To Buy: Cinnamon is readily available at most grocery stores, spice shops, and online retailers.

Cautions: While cinnamon is generally safe, check that you do not have an allergy if you have never used it.

Tips: Buy ceylon cinnamon as this is reported to be the best type to use.

Clove

Properties & Claimed Health Benefits:

- One of the strongest antioxidants known
- May help protect against cancer
- Can kill bacteria
- May improve liver health
- Can help regulate blood sugar
- May reduce stomach ulcers
- Used to improve circulation
- Clove oil is used for dental pain

Cloves are the flower buds of the clove tree, an evergreen that grows in India and Indonesia. It can be found in both whole and ground forms. Clove is a very strong antioxidant and antimicrobial. It has been used for centuries to improve circulation, for tooth pain, digestion, and in formulas for pain. Clove is STRONG and should be used in small amounts, generally in formulas.

Where To Buy: Cloves can be easily found in most grocery stores, both in whole and ground forms.

Cautions: While cloves are generally safe when used in culinary amounts, concentrated clove oil should be used sparingly and cautiously. Pregnant and breastfeeding women should consult their medical practitioner before using clove supplements.

Tips: You can simmer whole cloves in boiling water for 5–10 minutes to make a soothing cup of clove tea mixed with cinnamon and cardamom for a wonderful winter tea that will warm you and give you amazing health benefits. Add raw local honey or manuka honey if needed.

Cranberry (Vaccinium macrocarpon)
Properties & Claimed Health Benefits:
- Helps to prevent urinary tract infections
- High antioxidant levels
- Improve heart health
- Prevention of Stomach Ulcers

Cranberries are a member of the heather family and are related to blueberries, bilberries, and lingonberries. Cranberries are most often consumed as juice, which is normally sweetened and blended with other fruit juices. Unsweetened cranberry juice effectively prevents and is part of a treatment plan to treat urinary tract infections. Pure cranberry juice can be a good source of Iodine.

Where To Buy: Cranberries are readily available in most grocery stores, typically in fresh, dried, or juice form. You can also find cranberry supplements in health food stores or online.

Cautions: Although cranberry juice can be a very effective preventative and treatment for urinary tract infections, always seek medical advice for infection as it can lead to serious health implications.

Tips: If you suffer from recurrent urinary tract infections, try a shot of pure, unsweetened cranberry juice daily and drink plenty of fluids as a preventative.

Cream Of Tartar
Properties & Claimed Health Benefits:
- Alleviates muscle cramps and pain
- Can help with acid reflux
- Promotes balanced pH levels in the body
- May help reduce urinary tract infections

- Can assist in reducing the symptoms of gout
- Can help prevent yeast overgrowth after antibiotic use
- Relieves constipation
- Lowers blood pressure
- Used in cooking to stabilize egg whites and make meringue
- Used in a famous 'adrenal formula'

Cream of tartar is a baking ingredient that has been found to have some amazing health benefits. Some have science behind them, and many are anecdotal. But this wine-making by-product is an amazing item to have handy in your cupboard.

Where To Buy: Cream of tartar is readily available in most grocery stores, baking supply stores, and online retailers.

Cautions: High intakes of cream of tartar may lead to hyperkalemia or dangerously high blood potassium levels due to its high potassium content.

Tips: Start with ⅛ of a teaspoon and go up from there. Ensure you never use too much and consume plenty of salt to counter the high potassium in this product.

Dandelion

Properties & Health Benefits:
- Nutrient-rich leaves can be eaten or juiced
- A well-known liver detoxer
- Anti-inflammatory action
- Natural potassium sparing diuretic
- Rich in antioxidants
- Supports immune system
- May help to regulate blood sugar levels
- Helps to lower blood pressure

- Reduce cholesterol and triglyceride levels
- Has 'bitter' qualities and supports healthy digestion

The dandelion is often dismissed as a stubborn weed; however, people have used dandelion flowers, leaves, and roots as food and for medicinal purposes for centuries in tinctures, teas, and vinegars to support digestion, liver health, heart health, and more.

Where To Buy: Dandelion leaves and roots can be picked from your own backyard or purchased at health food stores.

Cautions: While dandelion is generally safe for most people, it can cause allergies in some individuals. Exercise caution if you have allergies to related plants like ragweed, marigolds, or daisies. Also, if you have any medical conditions or are taking medications, consult your medical practitioner before using dandelion.

Tips: When foraging for dandelion leaves, collect them from areas free of pesticides and other contaminants. Start with small doses if you're new to dandelion to see how your body responds. Consider consulting an herbalist or medical practitioner for personalized guidance.

Elderberries (Sambucus)
Properties & Health Benefits:
- High in Vitamin C
- Supports respiratory and lung health
- Can be used for sore throats and coughs
- High antioxidant power
- Promotes heart health
- Lowers inflammation
- Boosts your immune system - science-backed.
- Good for blood sugar management

Elderberry is one of the most common medicinal plants in the world. It has been used in folk medicine to treat fever, rheumatism, sciatica, infections, and more. Today, elderberry supplements are mainly used to treat cold and flu symptoms.

Where To Buy: Elderberries can be found in various forms, such as dried, syrup, or supplement capsules. They are available at health food stores, herbal shops, and online retailers.

Cautions: Some varieties of elderberries can be toxic in their natural state and should always be cooked or processed before consumption or simply buy a prepared supplement

Tips: Elderberry syrup or tea is a popular and delicious way to incorporate elderberries into your daily routine. It has been proven to help reduce the chances of catching colds and flu and help reduce their severity and duration if you catch them.

Fennel Seeds (Foeniculum vulgare)
Properties & Claimed Health Benefits:
- Combats bad breath
- Improves digestion
- May help to regulate blood pressure
- Supports the lungs for people with respiratory ailments
- Improves skin appearance
- Purifies blood
- Traditionally used to improve eyesight
- Reduces Gas

Fennel is an aromatic culinary herb and medicinal plant. Fennel plants are green and white, with feathery leaves and yellow flowers. Both the crunchy bulb and the fennel plant seeds have a mild, liquorice-like flavor. Yet, the flavor of the seeds is more potent due to their powerful essential oils.

Where To Buy: Fennel seeds are readily available in most grocery stores and health food shops in whole and ground forms.

Cautions: Although eating fennel and its seeds is likely safe, consuming higher doses in supplement form may react with certain medications and is unsafe for pregnant women. Check with your medical practitioner before use.

Tips: Fennel seeds can be used in many ways like all spices, but you can simply chew some seeds after a meal (Indian restaurants sometimes offer Fennel seeds but more often offer customers mints these days), and they will help with bad breath, digestion, and gas.

Garlic (Allium sativum)

Properties & Claimed Health Benefits:

- Used to prevent and recover from the common cold and other infections
- Improves circulation and heart health
- Active compounds can reduce blood pressure
- Improves cholesterol levels,
- Traditionally said to help you live a longer life!
- May help detoxify heavy metals in the body
- Increase libido

Garlic contains compounds with potent medicinal properties. Hippocrates, the father of medicine, prescribed garlic for his patients and used it to treat many medical conditions. Garlic is rich in sulfur compounds; this is believed to be responsible for the taste and scent of garlic and its medicinal properties.

Where To Buy: Garlic is readily available in most grocery stores as fresh bulbs or pre-minced or powdered forms. You can also find it in various dietary supplements.

Cautions: Garlic can interact with certain medications, especially blood thinners. Consult your medical practitioner before consuming large amounts of garlic, particularly if you're on medication. Some individuals may experience digestive discomfort or heartburn when consuming garlic.

Tips: Garlic can be used in raw form, cooked form, or even in powder and capsule form, and I have found them all to be useful. Fresh garlic cloves can be crushed and added to a glass of milk and taken at least once daily as a traditional remedy for colds and flu. For full health benefits from raw garlic, crush it and leave it to oxidize for three minutes before using. This allows two compounds in garlic to mix and create magic!

Gelatine

Properties & Health Benefits:

- Source of collagen
- A common remedy to improve hair and nail strength
- Improves joint health
- Improves gut health
- Supports digestion of other foods
- Improves skin health and appearance
- Muscle recovery
- Improves bone health
- Can improve sleep quality due to its unique amino acid profile

Gelatin is protein-rich and has a unique amino acid profile with many potential health benefits. There is evidence that gelatin may reduce joint and bone pain, increase brain function, and help reduce the signs of skin aging. Because gelatin is colorless and flavorless, it's super easy to include in your diet. You can make gelatin at home by following a simple recipe or buying it pre-prepared to add to your everyday food and drinks.

Where To Buy: When looking to buy it in grocery stores or online, you'll likely come across gelatin in the form of sheets, granules, or powder. Also, you can use collagen peptides, a popular supplement that can be added to shakes and doesn't turn into jelly, but this is more expensive.

Cautions: Gelatin is generally well-tolerated; opt for grass-fed or pasture-raised products to avoid artificial hormones, antibiotics, and GMOs. Gelatine can NOT be used as a sole source of protein as it lacks essential amino acids.

Tips: Studies have shown that taking gelatin 30 minutes before exercise reduces the amino acids needed for joint repair. This confirms an age-old folk tale that eating specific foods aids in repairing the corresponding organ or part of your body. For example, consuming muscle meat is best for muscle growth, while eating collagen supports your body's collagen (skin, joints, bones, etc.).

Ginger (Zingiber officinale)
Properties & Health Benefits:
- Boosts immune system health
- Fights inflammation and infections
- Aids digestion
- Can help to lower cholesterol
- Supports heart health
- Fights free radical damage
- Promotes detoxification
- Helps to improve skin health
- May Aid weight loss
- Improves mood and energy levels
- Supports Respiratory Health
- Helps the body balance blood sugar levels

Ginger is a powerhouse of healing! Ginger is probably best known for helping with morning sickness, but this is one of the lower-level things that it does. A great anti-inflammatory, pain reliever, digestive aid, and circulation improver, ginger can be used in dry powder form, fresh form, in tea, juiced, and tinctured. It is very versatile and should be used regularly by most people, especially those over 40!

Where To Buy: United States - any grocery store. United Kingdom – any supermarket or convenience store

Cautions: Peel non-organic ginger, and be careful not to over-consume, especially if pregnant or on blood thinning medication

Tips: Ginger is powerful and works, so small doses to start is a must.

Goji Berry (Lycium barbarum)

Properties & Claimed Health Benefits:

- Are an adaptogen
- High levels of beneficial plant compounds help protect the heart
- Supports the circulatory system
- Helps in lowering bad cholesterol levels
- Improves immune function
- Antioxidant-rich
- High carotenoids that help protect the retina in the eye
- Anti-ageing properties
- Help in lowering blood sugar levels
- Helps to detoxify the liver
- Promote healthy skin
- Mood and energy booster
- Boosts fertility

Goji berries have been used for centuries in China. They are known for their sour flavor. In addition to their vitamins, minerals, and antioxidant content, these berries may promote immune function, eye health, heart health, and liver function. They're available in several forms and can be added to numerous recipes.

Where To Buy: Goji berries are available in health food stores, online retailers, and some grocery stores. Look for organic and high-quality options.

Cautions: People allergic to goji berries should refrain from having them. Those allergic to nightshades, nuts, peaches, or tobacco may also be allergic to goji berries. It is advised to consult your medical practitioner before consuming goji berries if you suffer from allergies.

Tips: Goji berries can be consumed as supplements, eaten dried (raw or cooked), added to herbal teas and soups, or enjoyed as goji berry juice. 1 ounce a day is said to be a good amount to eat or make into an infusion.

Grapefruit (Citrus paradisi)
Properties & Health Benefits:

- Rich in Vitamin C
- May help prevent insulin resistance and diabetes
- The flavonoids (the white stuff around it when you peel it) improve Vitamin C action in the body
- Benefits your immune system
- Has weight loss benefits
- Reduces the risk of kidney stones
- Rich in antioxidants
- Heart-healthy
- Boots skin health

Grapefruit is a tropical citrus fruit known for its sweet yet tart taste.

It is rich in nutrients, antioxidants, and fiber. This makes it one of the healthiest citrus fruits you can eat.

Where To Buy: You can find grapefruit at most grocery stores or farmers' markets; it is readily available year-round.

Cautions: While grapefruit offers numerous health benefits, it can interact with certain medications, including statins and blood pressure. Grapefruits can interfere with the liver's ability to break down medications, so please consult your medical practitioner if you have concerns about potential interactions.

Tips: Enjoy grapefruit as a snack or in salads for a refreshing burst of flavor. You cannot eat the peel, but the 'pith,' the white stuff under the peel, is great for artery health and allows vitamin C to do more work in the body.

Hawthorn (Crataegus monogyna)

Properties & Health Benefits:

- The berries, leaves, and flowers can be used as medicine
- May have anti-aging properties
- Used to aid digestion
- Reduce blood cholesterol levels
- Lower blood pressure
- Anti-inflammatory properties
- Loaded with antioxidants
- Used traditionally to reduce anxiety
- Traditional herbal medicine used to treat heart failure

Hawthorn (crataegus species) is touted by many herbalists to be the perfect herb for the heart. It has been used to treat heart disease since the 1st century. By the early 1800s, American doctors were using it to treat circulatory disorders and respiratory illnesses. Traditionally, the berries were used to treat heart problems ranging from irregular heartbeat, high blood pressure, chest pain, hardening of the arteries, and heart failure. The leaves and flowers are used medicinally.

Where To Buy: Hawthorn may be difficult to find at your local grocery store. However, you may be able to find it at farmers' markets and specialty health food stores or online (See Resources page for my recommendation).

Cautions: Many herbalists use hawthorn with patients on heart medication to help reduce the need for the medication. I would suggest that if you are on medication, you speak with your medical specialist or an herbalist who is willing to help, take responsibility, and collaborate with your doctor.

Tips: Hawthorn is available in non-standardized and standardized capsules, liquid extracts, tinctures, and solid extracts. A bitter-tasting tea can also be made from dried hawthorn leaves, flowers, and berries. I find that a tincture is the most convenient way to take hawthorn 2 to 3 times daily.

Honey

Properties & Health Benefits:

- Natural sweetener.
- Rich in antioxidants.
- Supports the immune system.
- Helps heal wounds when applied topically.
- Soothes sore throats and coughs.
- Aids digestion and reduces bloating.
- Good for the skin as a natural moisturizer.
- Common in homemade cough remedies.
- Quick energy boost.
- May provide allergy relief.

- Can assist in weight management.

Honey is a versatile and natural ingredient that offers various health benefits. It has been used for centuries for its nutritional and medicinal properties.

Where To Buy: Honey is widely available, but local farmers' markets are the best places to buy. You can choose from a variety of types, including raw honey, manuka honey, and more.

Cautions: While honey is generally safe, it should not be given to infants under one year old due to the risk of botulism. Diabetic individuals should use honey in moderation and monitor their blood sugar levels.

Tips: When buying honey, consider opting for local, raw, unprocessed honey for the maximum health benefits.

Honeygar

Properties & Health Benefits:

- Used in folk medicine against infections such as cystitis (in cows and people)
- Used by D. C Jarvis for arthritis
- Used by D. C Jarvis for asthma
- May help to alleviate seasonal allergies and cold symptoms
- Traditionally said to improve heart health
- Helps in the digestion of food
- May help blood sugar regulation (especially if mixed with spices such as Cinnamon)
- Acetic acid within it may promote weight loss
- Improves skin health
- Anti-inflammatory properties
- Helps in detoxification
- Energy boosting

Honey and vinegar have been used for medicinal and culinary purposes for thousands of years, with folk medicine often combining the two as a health tonic. I have a book worth reading from D. C. Jarvis, who writes of his experiences with 'honeygar,' using it to treat everything from cystitis in cows to asthma, arthritis, rheumatism, colds, flu, and more! The mixture, typically diluted with water, is thought to provide a range of health benefits, including weight loss and reduced blood sugar levels.

Where To Buy: Honeygar can be found in most health food stores, online retailers, and even at home by mixing raw honey and apple cider vinegar in the desired ratio.

Cautions: If you have allergies to honey or apples, it's important to be cautious when using Honeygar. Consult with your medical practitioner before adding honeygar to your diet, especially if you have underlying health conditions or are on medication.

Tips: Honeygar is best drunk regularly, three times per day, for treating an issue. 1 tablespoon in a glass of warm water works well, but be careful not to ruin your teeth.

Horsetail (Equisetum)

Properties & Health Benefits:

- Used by herbalists to promote bone growth
- Supports nail and hair growth.
- Promotes wound healing.
- Provides joint and muscle support
- Supports urinary tract health and alleviates urinary tract infection symptoms.
- Assists in detoxification with its diuretic properties.
- Used to improve skin health.
- Eases respiratory conditions like bronchitis and asthma.
- Traditionally used for digestive issues and upset stomach.

- Rich in antioxidants

Horsetail is an ancient fern that has been used as an herbal remedy since the Greek and Roman Empires. It's believed to have multiple medicinal properties. It has traditionally been used to treat wounds and bone health and promote hair and skin health.

Where To Buy: The best place is to purchase online (See Resources page for my recommendation)

Cautions: Pregnant and breastfeeding women, people with kidney disease, and those who take antiretroviral drugs should seek advice from their medical practitioner before consuming them.

Tips: Added to nettle and oat straw, herbalists have long used horsetail to help people with osteoporosis.

Jasmine (Jasminum)

Properties & Claimed Health Benefits:

- Used to relieve stress
- High in antioxidants
- Can be used to help improve sleep quality in anxious people
- May help to protect your heart
- Could boost brain function
- May protect against Alzheimer's and Parkinson's disease
- Can help to lower your risk of type 2 diabetes

Jasmine is a fragrant flower with a wide array of properties and health benefits. It is known for its stress-relieving and anxiety-reducing properties. It has also been used traditionally to enhance sleep quality and promote restful nights.

Where To Buy: You can find jasmine products, including essential oils, teas, and skincare items, at health food stores, online retailers, and specialty botanical shops.

Cautions: While generally safe, jasmine essential oil should be used in moderation. Some individuals may be sensitive to it. Always perform a patch test before applying it to your skin. If you are pregnant or have a medical condition, consult with your medical practitioner before use.

Tips: Jasmine can be used with other calming herbs, such as chamomile, 60 to 30 minutes before bed to help aid in a restful night's sleep.

Kefir

Properties & Claimed Health Benefits:

- Probiotics within can improve gut health
- More powerful probiotic than yogurt
- Potent antibacterial properties
- Great source of protein and many vitamins
- Promoted to protect against cancer
- May be able to be consumed by lactose-intolerant people
- May reduce blood pressure
- Improve bone health and lower the risk of osteoporosis

Kefir is a cultured, fermented milk drink. It is like yogurt but thinner in consistency, making it more suitable for drinking. Due to carbon dioxide, Kefir has a tart, sour taste and a slight fizz, a by-product of the fermentation process.

Where To Buy: You can find kefir in most grocery stores or health food stores, often in the European or Eastern European section.

Cautions: While kefir is generally safe for most people, those with severe lactose intolerance or dairy allergies should opt for non-dairy alternatives.

Tips: Drink kefir on its own first thing in the morning for a probiotic and deep nutritional start to the day. You can buy Kefir 'grains' that you place in milk, and they produce kefir for you. This produces the best kefir with any strains of good bacteria and yeasts.

Leek (Allium ampeloprasum)
Properties & Health Benefits:

- Lower blood pressure levels
- Fight infections
- Contains a variety of nutrients
- Diuretic properties
- May reduce inflammation and promote heart health
- Packed with beneficial plant chemicals
- May aid in weight loss
- May protect against certain cancers

The leek is a relative to onion and garlic. Like garlic and onion, leeks have a plethora of health benefits and should be incorporated into your diet regularly.

Where To Buy: You can find fresh leeks in the produce section of most grocery stores. They are commonly available in many regions, especially during the fall and winter. They are easy to grow, so give them a try!

Cautions: Leeks are generally safe to consume. However, if you have allergies to related plants like garlic or onions, consult your medical practitioner before adding leeks to your diet.

Tips: Buy organic and try using leeks in soups, broths, juice and boiled (keep the water)

Lemongrass (Cymbopogon citratus)
Properties & Health Benefits:

- High in antioxidant
- Anti-viral properties

- Antimicrobial properties
- Anti-inflammatory properties
- May help regulate your cholesterol
- Can help you relax and destress
- May help promote healthy digestion
- May act as a diuretic
- May help reduce high systolic blood pressure
- Has been used to help relieve symptoms of premenstrual symptoms

Where To Buy: You can sometimes buy lemongrass in grocery stores, but I buy plants from the garden center and grow them myself. It is part of the mint daily, is hardy, and grows fast.

Cautions: Lemongrass may interfere with thyroid medication, so get advice from your medical practitioner before taking it in large doses.

Tips: Lemongrass has an amazing aroma. Try making tea, crushing the leaves, and taking a whiff, and you will immediately begin to relax.

Linden (Tilia Americana)

Properties & Health Benefits:

- Can help reduce anxiety and insomnia
- Promotes relaxation and reduces stress
- Provides antioxidant benefits
- Supports respiratory health
- Soothes the digestive system
- Can relieve headaches and migraines in some people
- World-famous cold and flu remedy
- Supports cardiovascular health
- Alleviates muscle tension

Another beautifully smelling herb, linden can be used in large doses.

Linden is one of the world's most widely used cold and flu remedies. It is high in antioxidants, soothes the gastrointestinal tract, and supports lung health. Linden is also an herb that helps relax the nervous system, promoting a calming effect. If that's not enough, Linden also positively impacts the heart. This is why it is part of my regular daily infusions.

Where To Buy: I buy linden in bulk and use it in 1oz amounts. (See Resources page for my recommendation)

Cautions: Linden should be taken away from medication as it may interfere with absorption.

Tips: A cup of warm linden and lemongrass infusion with manuka honey, drunk before bed at the onset of a cold, can, in my experience, help alleviate symptoms by the morning.

Marshmallow Root (Althaea officinalis)

Properties & Health Benefits:

- Used to relieve coughs and sore throats
- Used in herbalism to repair the gut lining
- Supports overall skin health
- Can help to fight infections
- Used in herbalism for years to treat issues with the urinary tract
- Supports heart health
- Can help ease congestion
- Aids in wound healing
- Helps to relieve skin irritations

Marshmallow root has been used for thousands of years to treat digestive, respiratory, and skin conditions. Its healing powers are due in part to the mucilage it contains.

Where To Buy: Marshmallow root can be purchased from herbal stores, health food shops, or online retailers specializing in herbs and natural remedies.

Cautions: It's generally safe for most people, but seek advice if you have allergies to other plants in the Malvaceae family (like hibiscus or okra). Pregnant and breastfeeding women should consult with their medical practitioner before using marshmallow root.

Tips: For topical applications, you can prepare marshmallow root in cold water and use it directly on the skin

Meadowsweet (Filipendula ulmaria)
Properties & Health Benefits:

- Anti-inflammatory
- Relieve Bronchitis
- Can be used for ulcers.
- Can be helpful in heartburn
- May be helpful for some painful conditions.
- Used to treat skin inflammation topically
- Can be used to help with upset stomachs
- Has been used as a diuretic
- Can be useful for joint inflammation

As part of the rose family, meadowsweet has been used as a diuretic in traditional medicine to alleviate joint pain and heartburn. It contains many compounds thought to have anti-inflammatory effects on the body.

Where To Buy: You can find meadowsweet in health food stores, herbal apothecaries, or online herbal retailers. (See Resources page for my recommendation)

Cautions: Used in small doses in teas and tinctures, meadowsweet is deemed safe, but in some rare cases, it can cause side effects. Therefore, many herbalists tend to advise starting with a small amount of tea. If there are no negative side effects, increase the dose slowly until you can comfortably take a full cup. If no adverse reactions are noticed, you should be fine with using larger doses, such as three cups a day.

Tips: Start with 1 tsp of dried herb and 300ml of hot water when making meadowsweet tea, and steep for 2 minutes. Increase the amount of herb and the time steeped gradually until you steep two teaspoons for 10-15 minutes for maximum benefits.

Milk

Properties & Health Benefits:

- Protein Powerhouse
- Used in many traditional Indian medicine remedies
- Packed with essential nutrients
- Supports proper immune system
- Rich source of calcium, phosphorus, and other minerals
- Good for muscle recovery
- Suggested for proper bone development in children

Milk is controversial today. It has been used for thousands of years in remedies, and in India (buffalo milk) is used as a delivery system. Goat's milk is nutritionally close to human milk and is still used by almost three-quarters of the world's population.

Where To Buy: Milk is widely available at grocery stores, supermarkets, and local dairies. I prefer raw milk from A2 cows fed grass all year round.

Cautions: Some people have a true milk allergy, although I don't know anyone with this condition. I do know some people who are lactose intolerant. In these cases, lactose-free milk, raw cow's milk, or goat milk can be substituted.

Tips: Try raw cow or goat milk from healthy animals. You may find it is a completely different experience from supermarket milk.

Nettle Leaf (Urtica dioica)

Properties & Health Benefits:

- Said to make bones strong and arteries flexible
- Used in herbalism to treat eczema
- Traditionally used to help manage arthritis
- Used to stimulate hair growth
- Treat disorders of the kidneys and urinary tract
- May help to control blood sugar in patients with diabetes
- Prevent or treat diarrhea
- Used for relief of asthma
- Speeds the healing of wounds
- Can be useful to help with anemia

This common weed that packs a sting could be the world's most nutritious plant! Forget all the superfoods you read about; nettle leaf is an amazing nutrient-dense plant ideal for use in daily nutritional herbal infusions.

Where To Buy: Nettle leaf can be found in health food stores, herbal apothecaries, or online retailers, but you can simply go out in the garden and cut, dry, and then use it in infusion.

Cautions: Be cautious when handling fresh nettle leaves as they may cause skin irritation due to their tiny stinging hairs. Cooking or drying the leaves eliminates this issue.

Tips: Nettle leaf is one of the most nutritious plants possibly in the world. Buy in bulk and drink regularly.

Oatstraw (Avena sativa)

Properties & Health Benefits:

- Promotes relaxation and reduces stress
- Helps treat skin disorders

- Used to nourish the nervous system
- Used to enhance sexual health
- Maintain digestive health
- Used to improve blood sugar levels
- Can contribute to good heart health
- Improves immune system
- May help to improve brain function

Oat straw is a wonderful-tasting herb used as part of my rotation of nourishing herbal infusions. Human studies indicate it may improve older adults' brain function and heart health. With a long history as a nervous system nourishing herb, it also possesses the ability to relax the mind and improve sexual well-being.

Where To Buy: You can find oat straw in bulk online (See Resources page for my recommendation)

Cautions: If you have a gluten allergy, you may also have a reaction, so in these cases, please use with caution and seek advice from your medical practitioner if needed.

Tips: In my opinion, this herbal infusion is best served warm with a little honey.

Onion (Allium cepa)
Properties & Health Benefits:
- Supports proper circulation
- Promotes heart health
- Aids in digestion
- Supports the detoxification process in the body
- Has strong anti-inflammatory properties
- Helps regulate blood sugar
- Exhibits antimicrobial properties

- High levels of quercetin
- May have anti-cancer potential
- Contains high antioxidants

From Greek athletes to modern scientists, onions have been revered for their health benefits for centuries. Containing similar healthy compounds to garlic and leeks, onions contain good amounts of vitamins and minerals, as well as compounds such as quercetin. Sulphur is another very important compound found in onions, a fundamental nutrient the body needs to function.

Where To Buy: Onions are readily available in most grocery stores, making them an easily accessible and affordable addition to your meals. Even organic onions are cheap.

Cautions: Onions are amazing for health and a powerful ally in retaining health, but they are also very powerful medicine. If juicing, start with very small amounts.

Tips: Boil, sauté, steam, eat raw and juice onions. They contain so many good benefits; get them every way you can!

Passionflower (Passiflora incarnate)

Properties & Health Benefits:

- May help reduce the effects of menopause
- Helps lower blood pressure
- Can reduce anxiety
- Helps address ADHD symptoms
- Helps reduce insulin levels
- Can improve sleep
- Reduces inflammation
- May calm your mind
- Soothe your stomach

The chemicals in passionflower have calming effects and have been traditionally used to help with sleep.

Where To Buy: You can find passion flower herbs online. Passionflower can also be grown at home if you have a green thumb and enjoy gardening. (See Resources page for my recommendation)

Cautions: While passionflower is generally considered safe, it may cause drowsiness in some individuals. It's advisable not to operate heavy machinery or drive after consuming Passionflower, especially if you're new to it.

Tips: Start with a low dose of passionflower and monitor your body's response. Gradually increase the dosage as needed.

Pineapple (Ananas comosus)

Properties & Health Benefits:

- Rich in vitamin C
- Contains high levels of anti-inflammatory and protein-digesting enzymes
- Contains antioxidants
- Can be used to aid digestion
- High in nutrition
- May boost immunity
- May speed recovery after surgery or strenuous exercise
- Contains manganese, essential for bone health
- High beta-carotene
  - May boost mood and energy levels

Pineapple is a tropical fruit known for its sweet and tangy flavour. It is not only delicious but also packed with health benefits. Juiced or eaten fresh, pineapple can aid in the digestion of proteins. Taken on an empty stomach, the enzymes are said to enter the body and do good work breaking down unwanted proteins.

Where To Buy: Pineapples are readily available in most grocery stores.

Cautions: Some people have allergies to pineapple. This is rare, but please make sure you aren't allergic before juicing large amounts.

Tips: When selecting a ripe pineapple, look for one firm with a sweet aroma and golden-yellow color.

Prunes (Prunus domestica)

Properties & Health Benefits:

- Helps constipation
- Helpful for overactive bladder
- High in potassium
- High in vitamins
- Can help to strengthen bones
- May help reduce cholesterol levels
- May help lower blood pressure
- Contains good amounts of antioxidants
- Supports a healthy gut microbiome

Prunes are well known to help with constipation, especially prune juice, but they are much more than that. With high nutrient and plant compound content, they are a wonderful treat.

Where To Buy: Prunes are widely available at grocery stores, health food stores, and online retailers.

Cautions: Possible side effects of prunes and prune juice include gas, bloating, and the risk of digestive upsets. Prunes are also high in purines, so people who suffer from gout should not drink the juice or eat too much.

Tips: Drinking plenty of water when consuming prunes can enhance their digestive benefits.

Red Wine

Properties & Health Benefits:

- Rich in antioxidants
- Shown to lower bad cholesterol
- Helps to keep a heart-healthy
- Increases blood circulation

It is challenging to make a case or a 'health benefits profile' for any alcohol. However, as most people know, moderate red wine intake may have some health benefits. Is it the nitric oxide it induces in the body? Antioxidants? Relaxation? Who knows, and the ongoing debate on how much is good vs. bad continues. We use small amounts that will have no negative effects on our bodies.

Where To Buy: Pretty much everywhere!

Cautions: Non-alcohol extracts are sometimes better for children or people who are recovering from alcohol addiction.

Tips: Cheap red wine works for extracts, but go for 12% volume or higher.

Rosemary(Salvia rosmarinus)

Properties & Health Benefits:

- High in antioxidants
- Contains impressive amounts of anti-inflammatory compounds
- Can have a blood pressure 'balancing effect'
- Can help fight infection in the body
- May improve your mood and memory
- Has a beneficial effect on the circulatory system
- Used in traditional herbal medicine to support brain health

- May protect vision and eye health
- Has shown heart health benefits
- May help to control blood sugar
- Improves digestion
- Has been used to promote healthy hair

Rosemary has been used for health going back centuries. Modern science backs up the use of rosemary for the brain, circulation, antimicrobial effects, antioxidant effects, and much more. This wonderful herb can be taken as a simple tea, tincture, or essential oil. All forms have benefits.

Where To Buy: You can find fresh or dried rosemary at most grocery stores or local markets. Alternatively, you can grow your own rosemary at home.

Cautions: Rosemary may exert effects like those of certain drugs used to treat high blood pressure, increase urination, and improve circulation. If you're on medication, consult your medical practitioner before adding rosemary tea to your diet.

Tips: Making rosemary tea at home is an easy way to control its strength and content. It can be bitter on its own; often, I mix it with mint, thyme, and lemon balm.

Schizandra

Properties & Health Benefits:

- Improves circulatory system
- Works as an adaptogen
- Effective against liver diseases
- Used in China for wheezing cough
- Can help balance blood sugar
- Antidepressant effect
- Adaptogenic properties

- Nervine properties

Schizandra chinensis (five-flavor fruit) is a fruit-bearing vine. Its purple-red berries are described as having five tastes: sweet, salty, bitter, pungent, and sour. It is a wonderful adaptogen, positively affecting the body, and can be used long-term.

Where To Buy: You can find schizandra in various forms, including dried berries, powders, and tinctures, at health food stores, herbal shops, and online retailers.

Cautions: Doses that are too high can result in gastric distress symptoms, such as heartburn. Schizandra can be drying, so it is best to consume some additional liquids when supplementing with this herb.

Tips: Schisandra berries and goi berries are a great combination to boost the whole body, with science-backed research showing positive effects on almost every main organ system.

Slippery Elm Powder (Ulmus rubra)

Properties & Health Benefits:

- Soothes and protects the gastrointestinal tract
- Can help Aid in the management of irritable bowel syndrome
- Eases digestive discomfort
- Supports respiratory health
- Relieves symptoms of acid reflux
- May help with food poisoning symptoms
- Can promote wound healing
- Reduces inflammation
- Used traditionally to help soothe the throat and mucous membranes
- Offers relief from skin irritations
- Can help with the relief of constipation

Slippery elm is a well-known herb for treating inflammation of the digestive tract. Its slippery, gooey nature can be off-putting for many people, but this is a big mistake as it is one of nature's best healers for the digestive tract.

Where To Buy: It can be found in most natural food stores. It can be used as a tea, as lozenges, in powder form, or in tablets.

Cautions: Pregnant or breastfeeding individuals should consult their medical practitioner before using slippery elm.

Tips: People on medications should not take slippery elm for two hours on either side of taking the medication as it may affect absorption.

Systemic Enzymes

Properties & Health Benefits:

- Reduces inflammation
- Supports digestive health
- Enhances immunity
- Improves blood flow
- Pain relief
- Detoxification
- Promotes the health of skin
- Boost mood and energy levels

Systemic enzymes are a group of enzymes that play a crucial role in various physiological processes. These enzymes work throughout the body to support overall health and well-being. I use Dr Wong's brand as they are the most potent I have found. Dr Wong is one of the world's leading experts on enzymes and has amazing testimonials for his product.

Where To Buy: Systemic enzymes are available in various forms, including supplements and capsules. They can be purchased at health food stores and online retailers. (See Resources page for my recommendation.)

Cautions: Check with your medical practitioner if you are taking blood thinning medication, as these enzymes also have a blood thinning effect.

Tips: Keep in mind that systemic enzymes work best when taken on an empty stomach for maximum absorption.

Thyme

Properties & Health Benefits:

- Can help lower blood pressure
- Strong antibacterial properties
- Can be used for Urinary tract and bladder infections
- Used to support the lungs and remedy coughs
- Can help boost immunity
- Essential oils in Thyme have strong disinfecting properties.
- Used to repel pests
- Can help to boost mood
- Helps to treat yeast infections

Thyme has been used by some of the great herbalists for hundreds of years. It is included in herbal mixtures for brain health, anti-infection, circulation, prevention of coughs, and so much more.

Where To Buy: Thyme is readily available in most grocery and health food stores or can be easily grown at home in a garden or pot.

Cautions: Thyme is generally safe when used in culinary amounts. However, individuals with allergies to the Lamiaceae family of plants. Other plans in this family include mint and basil, rosemary, lemon balm, and sage. If you react to any of these plants, you should be cautious and take advice from a professional practitioner.

Tips: Use thyme with onion and honey for a great kids' cough remedy.

Turmeric (Curcuma longa)
Properties & Health Benefits:

- Powerful anti-inflammatory properties
- Strong antioxidant properties
- Indian Ayurvedic medicine uses turmeric as a digestive aid
- Studies show it may help manage and prevent inflammatory bowel diseases
- Promotes heart health by reducing cholesterol levels
- Supports liver function and detoxification
- Used topically for skin conditions
- Supports joint health and is considered anti-arthritic
- Shows the potential to reduce the risk of neurodegenerative diseases
- Antibacterial and anti-viral properties
- Reduces the risk of heart disease

Turmeric is a golden spice with an impressive array of health benefits. Its active compound, curcumin, is known for its anti-inflammatory and antioxidant properties. Some herbalists believe that taking a curcumin extract rather than the whole herb is a mistake, as there have been studies to show the same anti-inflammatory effects in a turmeric product that had the curcumin removed.

Where To Buy: Turmeric is widely available in the fresh section of all grocery and health food stores. Buy organic NON-irradiated.

Cautions: Turmeric is generally safe for consumption, but rare allergic reactions, often after skin exposure, can lead to mild, itchy rashes. Use caution or seek advice from your medical practitioner if you have had your gallbladder removed or have gallstones. Also, it can stain, so you may wish to protect your work surfaces and wear gloves.

Tips: Mix with black pepper, ginger, and galangal and make a vinegar or tincture for a spicy superfood like nothing else.

Watercress (Nasturtium officinale)

Properties & Health Benefits:

- Recommended for heart health as it contains multiple heart-healthy compounds
- High antioxidant content
- Contains compounds that may help prevent certain types of cancer
- Used for bone health due to its calcium and vitamin K content
- Boosts Immune Function
- Nitrates found within it enhance circulation
- Contains high levels of carotenoids that may support eye health
- Can help to maintain healthy blood sugar levels

Watercress is a type of vegetable classified in the same family as kale, cabbage, and Brussels sprouts. It has a peppery flavor and many nutrients that support human health. Use it liberally in soups, salads, juice, and blended shakes.

Where To Buy: Watercress is often available in most grocery stores or local farmers' markets, particularly in the fresh produce section.

Cautions: While watercress is generally safe for consumption, individuals with certain medical conditions, like kidney stones, should consult their medical practitioner before consuming it in large quantities.

Tips: Always wash watercress thoroughly to remove any potential contaminants.

Yarrow (Achillea millefolium)

Properties & Health Benefits:

- Can be used to help treat urinary tract infections
- Wound healing

- Great for skin health, including acne
- Can stop bleeding
- Can help reduce symptoms of depression and anxiety
- Supports brain health
- Helpful for indigestion or heartburn.
- Acts as a diuretic to increase urine flow
- Helpful in amenorrhea (irregular menstrual cycle)
- May help with loss of appetite
- Can help reduce inflammation
- Fights infections

Yarrow is a common plant in the temperate regions of the world. Yarrow grows wild but is also cultivated for its lovely flowers. From a natural insect repellent to a pain reliever, infection fighter, and healing promoter, Yarrow is a herb everyone should keep around the home.

Where To Buy: You can buy dried yarrow or premade tea bags online or in various health stores. This herb also comes in other forms, such as tinctures, ointments, extracts, and powders.

Cautions: Yarrow is safe for most individuals. However, you should avoid it if you have a bleeding disorder, are pregnant, breastfeeding, undergoing surgery, or are allergic to ragweed.

Tips: Always source yarrow from reputable suppliers, and if harvesting in the wild, ensure you have proper identification and permission. A tincture is a good form to keep around; it's great to spray on a sore throat if you only have one.

Yogurt

Properties & Health Benefits:

- Enhances immune system function
- Supports gut health and digestion

- Aids in weight management
- Provides a good source of high-quality protein
- Contains essential vitamins and minerals, including B vitamins, potassium, and magnesium
- Has been shown to help lower blood pressure
- Can promote bone health due to its protein and calcium content
- Aids in the management of lactose intolerance

Yogurt is a popular dairy product made by the bacterial fermentation of milk. Yogurt is a popular breakfast for many people, and for a good reason, as it contains a healthy amount of protein, fats, and carbohydrates plus nutrients such as B vitamins and minerals plus gut healthy bacteria.

Where To Buy: Yogurt is readily available in most grocery stores, supermarkets, and dairy sections. It comes in various flavors and types. I prefer plain, full-fat, organic Greek yogurt

Cautions: If you have a milk allergy, you should avoid yogurt. If you are lactose intolerant, you may be OK with it.

Tips: Eating 1 cup of yogurt can provide almost half of your daily calcium needs. It also contains other vital nutrients.

Section 3

The 19 natural healing remedies

Traditionally, a 'remedy' is seen as a cure, something to address a current problem, so the term 'preventative' might not sound entirely accurate. However, I've included preventative natural healing remedies because of the modern world's exposure to an estimated 350,000 registered chemicals. In today's environment, providing our cells with the tools to function optimally is crucial.

These chemicals and toxins are relatively new to our world, and our bodies, while remarkable, must handle them with the same biological processes that existed when there were no man-made chemicals. Our bodies handle organic chemistry well, and our detoxification processes are adapting to new challenges. However, the quality and length of life are impacted by our environment. Some chemicals are proven to cause cancer, brain disorders, lung disorders, hormonal imbalances, and more.

To enhance our chances of avoiding chronic illness, nourishing our bodies is essential. Some estimate that our bodies need as many as 90 essential nutrients to function optimally — 16 vitamins, 2 (perhaps 3) essential fatty acids, 12 amino acids, and 60 minerals and rare earths. Consistent consumption of these nutrients is believed to provide our cells with everything they need to function correctly at any age.

Man-made chemicals require additional work in the human body, necessitating more nutrients to support the detoxification process. I strongly believe in optimizing plant-derived mineral intake for a healthy life and supplementing them accordingly. However, this book focuses on easy, quick, and affordable ways to improve health with food and herbs.

The following infusions are designed to nourish your cells, providing realistic doses of vitamins, minerals, amino acids, and plant compounds. These infusions support your cells in detoxifying, obtaining fuel, reducing inflammation, maintaining a robust immune system, and establishing a first line of defense against disease. They are safe for long-term use. In fact, herbalist Susan Weed recommends incorporating infusions into your daily routine, rotating them to ensure a good mix of nutrients and plant chemicals.

No Teas. I like tea, but tea is, on average, around 3 to 5 grams of a herb steeped in boiled water for around 3 to 5 minutes. You will definitely benefit from this, mostly from aromatic herbs, where you only need a small amount to benefit from the strong essential oils contained within them. However, nourishing infusions use 1oz / 30 grams of herb, steeped overnight. We never use aromatic herbs for these. This means you get all of the minerals, 500mg of calcium from Nettle infusion and 300 mg from oatstraw infusion, along with good amounts of other minerals such as magnesium, potassium, manganese, and many more. Also, the forms of minerals in herbal infusions are extremely absorbable and usable for your body, and you WILL feel a difference if you drink them regularly.

Preventative Daily Tonics

Remedy 1 - Infusions

To make an infusion (not a tea), we use 1 oz/30 grams of dried herb, weighed out and placed into a quart/1-liter glass container, such as a mason jar that can handle boiling water. I also use a large French coffee press to make them. Susan Weed doesn't like this method, but I find it works. Boil the kettle and pour straight over the herb to the top of the container (never plastic; make sure you have a jar designed to take boiling water, or it will crack). Stir with a wooden spoon or chopstick and cover.

Leave them for at least 4 hours or overnight. Strain and then refrigerate. I've had them in the back of a cold fridge for 3 days, and they have been OK, but they contain a decent amount of protein and can go off in that time, so aim to consume them in a day or two.

You can add a more fragrant herb to some if needed; sometimes, I use just a pinch of dried peppermint with nettle infusion. Play with it.

Nettle leaf - <u>For Adrenals, Energy, Strong Bones, Flexible Blood Vessels, Rebuilds Intestines, Helps with Arthritis and Is a Nutrition Powerhouse.</u>

A deep green to black-looking drink, you can see the nutrition in this drink, full of chlorophyll, a compound you could fill a book with all to itself, plus many minerals. In fact, here is a summary of Nettle from Susan Weed's website, which I cannot do better than: *"(Urtica dioica) builds energy, strengthens the adrenals, and is said to restore youthful flexibility to blood vessels. A cup of nettle infusion contains 500 milligrams of calcium plus generous amounts of bone-building magnesium, potassium, silicon, boron, and zinc. It is also an excellent source of vitamins A, D, E, and K For flexible bones, a healthy heart, thick hair, beautiful skin, and lots of energy, make friends with sister-stinging nettle. It may make you feel so good you'll jump up and exercise."* It's worth including in your daily routine, don't you think?

I prefer Nettle with a touch of mint, peppermint, or spearmint in it and served cold over ice. I rotate this in with every other infusion, so nettle, hawthorn, nettle, linden, nettle… Just because it is so full of nutrition and very helpful for the adrenals, gut lining, arteries, and bones.

Oat Straw - <u>For Libido, Relaxation, Nervous System Support, and Longevity</u>

Full of nutrition but not quite as much as nettle, yet both are densely nutritious with an overlap of nutrients, but they also differ. Oatstraw also contains steroidal saponins, which are said to nourish the pancreas and liver, improving digestion and stabilizing moods. It is also supposed to be a libido enhancer (I have never felt this effect. I believe it works more on people who have low libido due to stress) and is known as a longevity enhancer in Ayurvedic tradition.

Hawthorn Berry – <u>For Heart Health, Blood Pressure and Immune Support</u>

A truly amazing herb, hawthorn berries, leaves, and flowers all positively affect the heart, and you can use any of them for infusion. I choose the berries, or 'Haws,' which contain nutrition, amino acids, Vitamin D, B vitamins, Vitamins C, and more. But I believe this infusion is mostly used for its beneficial plant chemicals such as flavonoids, quercetin, vitamin X, rutin, choline, acetylcholine, and many more.

Regular use of hawthorn can

- Lower blood pressure
- Increase the effectiveness of the heart's pumping action
- Strengthen the heart muscle
- Slow the heartbeat
- Dilate coronary arteries
- Prevent heart disease, heart attack, and stroke
- Help those healing from heart surgery
- Support the immune system
- Increase longevity

As you can see, hawthorn berries are a true heart-specific remedy, traditionally used for many issues related to the heart, and modern science backs up those traditional uses. Certainly, it is an herb to use on regular rotation.

Goji Berry - Adaptogen, Eye Health, Ligament Health, Liver regenerator, Kidney and Heart strengthener, and capillary strengthener.

In traditional Chinese medicine, goji berries, also known as Lycium fruit, are used as a nutritive tonic for the liver, kidneys, and blood. They can be eaten 1oz daily as well as used as an infusion to strengthen weak muscles and ligaments, improve male sexual performance, and help relieve malnutrition (cachexia) usually associated with cancer or AIDS, according to Herbalist David Winston in his book on herbal adaptogens. High in carotenoids and flavonoids, goji berry can help stabilize the capillaries in the eyes traditionally, but this effect is also seen around the body with strengthened capillaries; circulation is improved, preventing varicose veins, spider veins, and cold hands and feet. Modern science backs up the hepatoprotective (liver protective) activity; it helps regenerate liver cells and protect against liver damage from medications.

Linden - the World's Leading Anti-Cold and flu remedy. Respiratory Tract Healer, Sore throat and Digestive tract soother, Anti-inflammatory, Anti-anxiety

Linden is a gentle yet powerful anti-inflammatory herb. Used for centuries as a remedy for colds and flu, linden contains nutrients, minerals, and vitamins. Like hawthorn, linden is mainly used for its plant chemicals to combat inflammation, colds & flu, aid the respiratory tract, and soothe gut issues. Safe for children, linden is one of the nourishing herbs you can reboil. Make it the usual way and strain. You can then add the herb to a pan of cold water, boil it, and leave it to cool. It will be quite slimy as it contains mucilage. These components of Linden are great for the respiratory and digestive tracts, soothing inflammation and encouraging healing. I like Linden very cold over ice or warmed with a little honey.

These are my favorite herbal infusions. You can find more information from Susan Weed (Website at the back of this book), but here are more herbs you can look into and swap into your rotation for their specific benefits or just to keep things interesting. Remember, though, these plants contain hundreds of nutrients and phytonutrients - chemicals that enhance our biology, improve our immune system, and create a stronger, healthy, and resilient YOU! With modern diets, we have lost touch with the wild plants we once consumed and evolved with, and these 'things' are missing from our lives for the most part.

My rotation

Nettle

Linden

Goji Berry

Hawthorn Berry

Other Herbs You can use

Burdock Root

Violet Leaf

Chickweed

Raspberry Leaf

Elder Flowers, Berries, and leaves

Plantain leaves

Marshmallow root

Slippery elm bark

Mullein stalk and leaf

Chickweed

Preventatives & Cures

In this section, you will find natural healing remedies that can serve as preventive measures and cures. Remember, we are using foods and herbs that are not drugs. They are much more complex than drugs. Therefore, you will find that one remedy will positively affect multiple issues, and it isn't just one remedy for one ailment. Also, because they are foods, they are safe to take to prevent disease as well as to cure them or make an illness pass faster and with fewer issues.

Bones, Joints, Tendons and Ligaments

<u>Remedy 2 - Bone Building Super Drink</u>

This bone-building super drink is a natural healing remedy number 2. After hearing how the rotation of nourishing herbal infusions had helped many women with osteoporosis and joint pain, I thought adding a mixed drink into the mix, taken daily or multiple times per week at least, should work faster. And lo and behold, it seems to work! Results seem to take some time, and anyone with osteoporosis should speak with a physical therapist who can help them incorporate proper exercise to improve their bones. Find a physical therapist who can tell you they have seen bone scans improve with previous patients. This means they know how to take you through the correct exercise to help remineralize bone. Athletes should consider this drink along with the daily infusions as it will help keep joints working correctly, and recovery from any unfortunate bone fractures will be repaired in quick time!

If you are already making and rotating the nourishing herbal infusions, you can simply add a tablespoon of horsetail to your nettle and/or oatstraw infusion when you make it.

When made, pour a large glass, put a pack or 1 tablespoon of gelatine in it and leave it for 30 to 60 minutes to allow it to 'bloom' or soak up water.

Then blend it for 5 minutes and enjoy.

If you are not drinking infusions (you should be) or if you have bone, skin, or hair issues, I suggest making this drink, as well as your regular infusions, a stand-alone one.

What you need:
- Suitable glass container
- ½ oz / 15 grams of dried Oatstraw
- ½ oz / 15 grams of dried nettle leaf
- 1 tablespoon of dried horsetail
- 1 litre of boiling water
- Half a pack or 1 tablespoon of gelatine

1. Place all the herbs into a suitable container
2. Pour over the boiling water and stir, then close the lid.
3. Leave overnight.
4. In the morning, strain the herbs and squeeze them to get everything out.
5. Place 250ml of the infusion into a pan
6. Add half a pack or 1 tablespoon of gelatine.
7. Let the mixture rest for 30 minutes and then gently heat the mix to

dissolve the gelatine OR, blend the mix and pour over ice (this is my preferred method, rather than heating it)

You can add dandelion leaf and/or alfalfa, two mineral-dense herbs, to help. But I have seen this basic mix work well over the course of a year. (It may have worked sooner, but people don't get scanned that often).

Remedy 3 - Sulphur Super Power Soup

This Sulphur Super Power Soup is great in addition to a daily rotation of herbal infusions and remedy number 2 – a bone-building super drink. This soup provides all of the nutrients bones and joints need to regenerate. It also offers a good amount of sulfur, which has an important role in building glucosamine and collagen, both integral to building healthy bones and joints, as well as supporting the immune system. If you might not be able to consume quite enough of the infusions, adding this soup as regularly as you can will help.

Step 1 - Broth Base

Make a broth with chicken carcasses or bones, whatever you have. It is good to use lots of cartilage, such as chicken feet, if you can get them (not everyone likes doing this), and meat on the bone is fine. You can also use any older vegetables you have, particularly the skins of vegetables, but only if they are organic and well-washed, of course, as you don't want a muddy broth. This is a rough and ready non-measure recipe. I used to wait until I had the right amount of bones, and that would mean hardly ever making the broth, so now, I use whatever I have; it's all good.

What you need:

- Large pot
- Chicken bones or carcasses
- Chicken feet (Optional)
- Old vegetables/peelings of vegetables
- Packet of Gelatine (Optional)

1. Fill your pot with whatever bones/ carcass you have.
2. Fill near to the top with water
3. Add a tablespoon of apple cider vinegar, and leave for 30 minutes
4. Bring to a boil and turn down to a simmer (or you could use a slow cooker)
5. Leave to simmer for at least four to six hours.
6. Add any carrots, onions, garlic, leeks, and celery you would like for the last two hours. Or you can just leave it as chicken broth, but if you have some vegetables, I would put some in for additional nutrition.
7. When done, strain out the bones and vegetables.

At this point, I generally add a packet of gelatine while it's still hot and then make the soup right away. This can be used as a base for any soup, sauce, gravy, etc.

Step 2 – Bone-building Soup

What you need:

- Large pot
- 1 tablespoon butter or coconut oil
- 1 chopped onion
- 1 leek trimmed, washed, and thinly sliced
- 1 large potato

- 225g /8oz of roughly chopped watercress
- 450ml / 16oz of the broth/stock you just made
- 450ml / 16oz quality milk
- Fresh ground black pepper or ground nutmeg to taste.
- A packet of gelatine (optional)

1. Heat a little butter, coconut, or your favorite oil in a pan.
2. Add the onion and leek. Cook over medium heat for 4 minutes or until softened, stirring occasionally.
3. Add the potato and watercress and cook for around 3 minutes or until the watercress is wilted.
4. Stir in the stock and milk. Simmer for around 20 minutes or until the potato is cooked. Stir occasionally
5. Remove from heat and allow to cool slightly before blending until smooth.

I have had people use this without or with an alternative milk, and all seem to work. I personally like to use full-fat, grass-fed raw milk. You may lose some benefit of this milk by heating it, but I know it's quality milk and great for bone building.

I like to add a packet or 1 tablespoon of gelatine to the finished soup. Not everyone does, and when it is heated, I think it's best served with some protein in it, but again, this is not necessarily needed. Remember, bone contains a large amount of protein structure into which the minerals are incorporated, so protein is important.

NOTE: Sulfur compounds are important for bones, joints, and ligaments. Fat-soluble vitamins A, D, and K2 are also very important for mineral absorption and to help minerals incorporate into bone. Sodium is also a key compound, so it is important to use a good Celtic-type sea salt that is a non-refined salt that contains all the micro-nutrients of the sea. Salt your food to taste.

Coughs, Colds & Flu and Lungs

Remedy 4 - Sweet and Spicy Tonic

This natural healing remedy is great for combating coughs and beating nasty bugs. It is circulation-stimulating and a brilliant digestive tonic.

I put this simple, sweet, and spicy tonic together after using each of the main ingredients in honey individually and seeing a similar Ayurvedic remedy.

Onions in honey is a traditional cough remedy, and if done well, it really works for both children and adults. Garlic in honey is a general 'immune booster' and antimicrobial, and ginger and honey are brilliant for coughs, circulation, and more. These are all great individually, but why not get all the benefits at once and then supercharge it?

What you need:
- 1 large jar (big enough for the below)
- 1 medium onion sliced thinly
- 1 bulb of garlic crushed and peeled and placed in whole
- 1 piece of ginger sliced, about the size of the bulb of garlic, larger if you have room
- 1 jar of (ideally) local, unpasteurized honey. Manuka honey works well, but it can be expensive.

1. Place the slices of onion in the jar.
2. Place the sliced ginger into the same jar.
3. Add the crushed garlic to the jar.
4. Completely cover all the ingredients with honey.
5. Tighten the lid of the jar and leave to sit for a couple of weeks.

You need to remember to undo the lid daily while it sits to 'burp' it. This is because it is fermenting and will create gas. Also, after burping daily, you can tip it upside down if you need to, ensuring you coat everything. Ideally, you should leave this mixture to sit for a couple of weeks.

I have tried this with cayenne pepper and chillies, but it was too hot for most people!

Use your sweet and spicy tonic straight from the jar. You can add a teaspoon amount to your favorite tea. Try picking the garlic out and eating it one clove at a time for an extra boost. You can keep topping this remedy up, so it should last long. This is now a sweet throat soothing, cough reducing, circulation stimulating natural healing remedy with strong anti-microbial activity.

Taking a spoonful daily as a preventative in the colder months is good. You can take it three times a day if a cold ensues, which will help bring it to an end. It will also aid digestion post-meal in warm water or in tea.

<u>Remedy 5 - Congestion Buster – Honey and Brandy will Make you Dandy!</u>

This congestion buster is a great one that comes from Tony Pantalleresco.

The natural healing remedy includes an essential oil, so I wasn't going to put this one in, but it works so well. I believe it should be on my list of 19 natural healing remedies. When you are congested and need to be clear-headed and able to breathe freely, this natural healing remedy will get you there.

What you need:

- 2 teaspoons of honey or your Sweet and Spicy Tonic mix (Natural Healing Remedy number 4 above)
- 1 teaspoon of brandy
- 1 to 2 drops of peppermint essential oil that states it can be taken internally.

1. Put your 2 teaspoons of honey or sweet and spicy remedy into a small glass.
2. Add the teaspoon of brandy.
3. Add a drop or two of peppermint oil.
4. Mix them up with a wooden spoon; it will become runny.
5. Close your eyes and knock it back.

You will feel the beneficial effects of the congestion buster natural healing remedy in seconds.

If you can't use brandy, you can substitute it for aloe vera juice.

If peppermint oil isn't available, you can use cayenne pepper instead. It makes it slightly different but will also open up your circulation and beat the congestion.

Remedy 6 – Breathe-easy - Nutraceutical POWER Juice

This breathe-easy natural healing remedy improves congestion and opens up airways and circulation. It reduces inflammation and has an abundance of antioxidants. It supports the immune system for viral infections and works to support the liver.

What you need to juice:

- 1 large red onion (or 2 small ones would work)
- 1 medium size grapefruit
- 1 chunk of ginger roughly 3 inches long (you add more or less to play with the dose).

1. Peel the onion and slice it to fit into the juicer.
2. Use a potato peeler to peel the grapefruit so you take off the outer skin but leave as much of the white piff as possible.
3. Peel and slice the ginger to fit into the juicer.
4. Push the onion and grapefruit through the juicer, then do the same with the ginger. This step will make you cry!
5. Pour the juice into a glass jar with a sealed lid and store it in the fridge.

As this is a strong natural healing remedy, I suggest starting with ½ teaspoon. Using too much of Breathe Easy, as it is potent, can cause dizziness. Once you get used to it, increase the amount up to 1 teaspoon and then gradually up to 1 tablespoon dose. You can use this natural healing remedy as often as you need to throughout the day to open up a congested chest, get your circulation going, and support your immune system to fight viral infections. Smokers tell me it helps clear their chests fast in the morning. Let me know how it works for you.

Remedy 7 - Honeygar Magic

Honegar magic is ideal for both dry and wet coughs. It can be used as a digestive aid and help control blood sugar. It is a great natural healing remedy for improving your circulation and preventing the onset of colds and flu.

What you need to blend:

- 1 pint of honeygar
- 1 large piece of ginger, about 6 to 8 inches
- 2 tablespoons of cinnamon

If you want to supercharge this natural healing remedy, you can add 1 teaspoon up to 1 tablespoon of cayenne pepper! The amount you use will dictate how potent your honegar magic becomes.

To adapt this remedy for bacterial infection or a more powerful circulatory benefit, add 2 to 8 cloves of garlic (crush and peel them before adding to the mixture).

1. Thinly slice the ginger.
2. Place all ingredients into a blender.
3. Blend on medium speed for 3 to 5 minutes.

To use your honeygar magic, take it in teaspoon amounts. You can add it to a small amount of water if that makes it easier to swallow. You can also gargle with this natural healing remedy, a great way to fight throat infections and mouth ulcers.

Stomach - Digestion, Acid Reflux, Bloating, Stomach Flu

<u>Remedy 8 - Stomach Fortifier</u>

Stomach fortifier is what I use to protect my gut from nasty bugs and to rebuild my microbiome from the use of antibiotics when I've needed them. Garlic does have antibacterial properties and may kill some of the beneficial bacteria and yeasts in the kefir. But it still seems to work to aid the gut.

This natural healing remedy works for all colds, flus, stomach bugs, and sore throats. Something I had forgotten about with the stomach fortifier is that it energizes me. Below is a full dose, but adjust the amounts to suit as this makes a large amount that is strong. I used a large, very aromatic bulb of garlic, which was almost too much for me. I'm a veteran of this natural healing remedy.

What you need to blend:
- 1 liter of yogurt or kefir
- 1 bulb of garlic (If this is your first time trying this remedy, you may want to use less garlic and work up to using a whole bulb).
- Glass jar with lid

1. Pour a pint of kefir or natural Greek yogurt into a blender.
2. Crush and peel one bulb (not just a clove) of garlic.
3. Leave the garlic to sit for 3 minutes before adding it to the blender.
4. Blend on medium for 5 minutes.
5. Pour as-is into a glass jar or strain any larger pieces of garlic that survived the blender out of the mix and then pour into a glass jar

with a lid.

6. Store in the fridge

Use the Simple Stomach Fortifier remedy in 1-tablespoon doses if you feel you have a gut bug coming in, suspect you might have eaten something dodgy, or are at the start of a cold or flu.

I have had people take a dose throughout the festive period, and they say it helps prevent getting colds and flus when mingling with lots of people. Be aware, though, that due to the large amount of garlic in this remedy, a side effect you may find is that you keep vampires away!

Caution - If you are on blood-thinning medication, please check with your medical practitioner, as garlic has a blood-thinning effect and can interfere with these types of drugs.

As I edit this book, we are deep into November. I have a child in nursery and one in primary school, both bringing home all the best bugs! Just this weekend, I made this natural healing remedy. At the start of the week, my wife came down with a tummy bug that the youngest had brought home from the nursery. Everyone then got this except me! I pushed my luck and lifted weights this week, and I've been working late and sleeping late. I have now got the sniffles and the start of a sore throat. I upped my dose of Stomach Fortifier to two tablespoons four times a day (luckily, I'm working from home), and the next morning... It was gone. Perfect timing for me to share this with you.

Remedy 9 - Acid Reflux Emergency Formula

Bicarbonate of soda and cream of tartar have been used on their own for many years as a natural remedy for acid reflux. I didn't think they would work together, but I think they work better as a pair than alone. I have added aloe vera juice with some people that needed an additional soothing effect, and it works well alongside these two ingredients to stop the discomfort.

What you need:
- ½ teaspoon of bicarbonate of soda or baking soda
- ½ teaspoon of cream of tartar
- 1 tablespoon aloe vera juice (optional)

1. In a small glass of warm water, mix the bicarbonate of soda or baking soda with the cream of tartar. Stir well for a minute.
2. Drink it down.

You could also add 1 tablespoon of aloe vera juice to the same mix. Some people find that it improves the results of this acid reflux emergency formula.

This is a quick and simple natural healing remedy that I put together for someone many years ago. They were using cream of tartar and salt with orange juice as an adrenal gland-supporting drink. I was at their house and suggested they mix the cream of tartar with bicarbonate of soda in a little warm water for some acid reflux she was having, as she didn't have any of the store-bought medication she usually used. This worked instantly; However, this is still only an emergency use remedy until you find the cause and cure of the indigestion.

Caution - Cream of tartar contains high amounts of potassium, so caution is needed. You should seek advice from your medical practitioner if you are on medication or have any kidney issues. The dose listed above should not be increased.

Remedy 10 - Indigestion / Acid Reflux Remedy

This natural healing remedy can be broken down into 4 different ways to help digest food more efficiently and prevent indigestion and acid reflux. This indigestion/acid reflux remedy also helps to support the liver and cleanse the blood. Some people have seen skin issues improve from continued use.

The 4 different ways:

Cup of Tea

Simply take:

- 10 grams of dandelion root
- 10 grams of burdock root
- 1 tablespoon of grated ginger root
- 2 teaspoons of apple cider vinegar (optional)

1. Place all the ingredients (except for the apple cider vinegar) into a pan with three cups of water.
2. Bring to a boil, then turn it down to simmer for 15 minutes.
3. Take it off the heat and leave to cool.

Start sipping slowly on half a cup pre-meal and finish the other half of the cup post-meal. This will greatly improve digestion and lessen bloating, indigestion, and acid reflux.

Some people like to add apple cider vinegar. If you want to try this tea, including the apple cider vinegar, follow the 3 steps above. However, add 1 to 2 teaspoons of apple cider vinegar directly into the mixture before you start drinking it. This seems to improve the formula for some people but can worsen acid reflux in others. Try without and then with and see how it goes for you.

Spoonful of Vinegar

Simply take:

- Glass jar with lid
- 10 grams of dandelion root
- 10 grams of burdock root
- 1 tablespoon of grated ginger root
- 250ml of apple cider vinegar
- 1 cinnamon stick

1. Place the dandelion root, burdock root, and grated ginger into a glass jar.
2. Cover with 250 ml of apple cider vinegar.
3. Either shake daily and wait 6 weeks or place in a blender, whiz it up for 10 minutes, and strain.

I like the traditional method but have done both. If you decide to shake and wait 6 weeks, add a stick of cinnamon to the jar.

Take one teaspoon to 1 tablespoon in a small amount of warm water pre-meal to help with digestion.

Sip of Digestive Wine

Simply take:

- Glass jar with lid
- 10 grams of dandelion root

- 10 grams of burdock root
- 250ml of dry red wine
- 1 cinnamon stick

1. Place the dandelion root and burdock root into a glass jar.
2. Cover with 250 ml of dry red wine.
3. Either shake daily and wait 6 weeks or place in a blender, whiz it up for 10 minutes, and strain.

Again, I like the traditional method but have done both. If you decide to shake and wait 6 weeks, add a stick of cinnamon to the jar.

Take one tablespoon to 1 ounce in a small amount of warm water pre-meal to help with digestion.

Pipet of Tincture

Simply take:

- Large glass container
- Dandelion root
- Burdock root
- Grated ginger root around 4 inches in size
- Bottle of Vodka or brandy

1. Fill the glass container to one-third full of a 50/50 mix of dried dandelion and burdock root.
2. Add the grated ginger.
3. Then, fill it with vodka or brandy.
4. Shake the container regularly for the next 6 weeks.
5. After six weeks, pour the tincture into its final container, straining out all the plant material.

If you do not want to wait 6 weeks, let the mixture soak for a day or two so that the hard roots become softer. Then, blend all the contents into a blender for 10 minutes. Once blended, pour and strain a small amount for immediate use, and pour the rest back into the original container to let it sit for six weeks. This allows for a stronger end product.

You can purchase little bottles used for tinctures quite cheaply; they have a pipet on top so you can measure out a few drops up to a dropper full. Remember to sterilize glass jars before using them.

There are lots of digestive bitter remedies out there; some throw in the whole kitchen sink, but I like to stick to simple herbs that work. Only a small amount of this natural healing remedy is needed, so this version is good to travel with. 1 drop into hot water before a meal can be amazing for some people. Make sure you swish over your tongue and around your mouth before swallowing. Suppose I'm having a heavy meal and I'm at home. In that case, I might add a dash of apple cider vinegar into the mix when the water has cooled down, and I sip it before, during, and after the meal.

This is a simple indigestion/acid reflux remedy, but it is a powerful one. Stomach issues are a huge problem all around the western world due to our diets and lifestyle. It also doesn't help that we have forgotten, for the most part, that we have utilized bitter herbs and foods for centuries. The whole digestive tract contains receptors for the bitter taste, usually from a chemical known as an Alkaloid contained within plants. Poisonous plants often contain alkaloids, so the effects we get from bitters - more stomach acid being produced and general 'preparedness' to process what's coming down the hatch, is thought to be a reaction to the potential poison. Guido Mase explains bitters beautifully in his book *Wild Medicine Solutions*.

Bonus Indigestion Remedy

Controversial Remedy (Do or Die?)

There are a lot of things that are much more controversial in life, I'll agree. But in the world of acid reflux, two ingredients, apple cider vinegar and cayenne pepper, seem to either work very well or cause issues. Look on the internet or use this with other people in a group and share your results. Some people will say, "It's amazing. It gets rid of stomach acid, indigestion, and bloating and even improves bowel movements." Others will say it worsened their reflux; the pepper was hot, etc. I use honeygar (honey mixed with apple cider vinegar) with cayenne. I feel this is a good winter-warming morning drink to get the intestines to wake up and warm up.

What you need:
- 1 tablespoon of honeygar
- Half a teaspoon of cayenne pepper

1. Mix together in a small glass of warm water and swallow for indigestion. This has worked amazingly for some people.

Remedy 11 - Protect and Soothe

This protect and soothe remedy is made from slippery elm and can be taken in 2 different ways.

Slippery elm is full of mucilage, which means it will thicken in water. I love it; some people don't like it, but this is THE herb for protecting and soothing your throat through your digestive tract. It is a wonderful herb and is indicated for soothing the upper respiratory, urinary, and digestive tract.

Drink - Slippery elm tea

You need:

- 1 cup of boiling water
- 1 teaspoon of slippery elm powder
- 1 teaspoon honey

1. Pour freshly boiled water into a cup
2. Stir the slippery elm powder into the water
3. Stir in the honey and allow it to cool and thicken for a few minutes.
4.
5. Sip the protect and soothe remedy slowly and enjoy the feeling as it slides down and coats all of your digestive tract.

Some people like to add lemon juice or cinnamon, but I like it as it is. I suggest you start simply and play from there. Let me know how you like it best.

Snack - Slippery elm balls

You need:

- 2 tablespoons of slippery elm powder
- 2 tablespoons of honey

1. Mix equal parts honey (ideally manuka or local raw honey, but any works) and slippery elm powder in a bowl.
2. Mix well until you have a consistency that allows you to make marble-sized balls. It should be quite a dry mixture.
3. Adjust the mixture as required to get the right consistency.
4. As you roll the small balls, roll them in some more slippery elm powder to coat them, and then place them into a container.

They are ideal to travel with. Pop a ball into your cheek and let it melt over time, slipping into your digestive tract and coating everything with a soothing, cooling protective layer. Take them with you and pop one anytime you need to.

Alternative Option

There is an alternative option for this Protect and Smooth remedy if slippery elm is not for you, and that is to use marshmallow root.

Drink

You need:

- Glass jar
- 1 oz of marsh mallow root
- 1 pint to 1 liter of room-temperature water

1. Pour the water into a glass jar
2. Add the marsh mallow root.
3. Shake and leave for a few hours or overnight.
4. It will make a slightly slimy mixture. You can usually refill it with water and get a therapeutic second batch from it.

Some people enjoy this cold and on its own; I like adding something to it. Cinnamon, cardamom, or vanilla - just a little of something to detract from the taste. I also like to have it warm, although I'll take a shot of it cold throughout the day.

Caution - The slippery elm and marshmallow root should be removed from medications as they may impair absorption.

Remedy 12 - Digestive Tea

A great all-rounder that tastes good, so people like to make this Natural Healing Remedy in batches and drink it several times per day. It soothes, helps bloat, improves digestion, helps indigestion, and lowers inflammation in the digestive tract. It has been known to help agitated people relax and aid their digestion. It also benefits the urinary tract and can help fend off bugs. This one contains more ingredients but is worth gathering, especially as you can make this digestive tea in larger batches for the whole family to enjoy throughout the day. It's a favorite at our house as a post-meal beverage for everyone, including guests, rather than coffee.

What you need:
- Large teapot
- 1 teaspoon of Chamomile flowers
- 1 teaspoon of Fennel Seeds
- 1 teaspoon of Meadowsweet
- 1 teaspoon of Marshmallow root finely chopped
- 1 teaspoon of Yarrow

1. Put the herbs and seeds in a large teapot
2. Bring a 500 ml / 16 fl oz of water to the boil and pour into the large teapot.
3. Let it sit for 10 minutes and serve.

You can take 250ml of this natural healing remedy two to three times per day. This digestive tea works wonders. I love the taste, which contrasts with many natural remedies that work. I have had feedback from many people that this solid all-rounder has helped cure acid reflux, stomach bloating, gas, constipation, general digestive discomfort, and more. Regularly using this natural healing remedy will help relieve issues, but its greatest power is possibly preventing future issues.

Alternatively, you can try sipping 150ml of the digestive tea before, during, and after a meal. Remember not to drink too much with a meal. Have a few small sips starting 15 minutes pre-eating, a few sips during, and finish the drink 30 minutes post-meal. This will aid the whole digestive process.

TIP: Buying these herbs in bulk means they last for a long time and are always there when you need them. But if this natural healing remedy is too much of a faff and your digestion is usually good, you can use chamomile and fennel seeds and still get great results. I travel with those two mixed herbs and take them as tea, which keeps my digestive tract running well.

1. Put the chamomile and fennel seeds in a teapot.
2. Bring a 500 ml / 16 fl oz of water to the boil and pour into the large teapot.
3. Let it sit for 10 minutes and serve.

Heart, Circulation, Brain, Eyes, and Nervous System

Remedy 13 - Heart Health Super Drink

I love the taste of this heart health super drink and find I drink it regularly. It is made with hawthorn berries, schizandra berries, and goji berries. They are best consumed daily to get the most benefit from each of the berries in this natural healing remedy. Each of these berries is amazing in its own right and has constituents that nourish just about every organ in the body.

Goji and schizandra are true adaptogenic herbs, meaning they are safe to consume for long periods. They positively affect the endocrine and nervous systems to help balance human biology. This may sound a bit general, but they have such a wide reach and really do help 'adapt' to stresses and the many stressors we have today. A great book to dive into in an understandable way would be Herbalist David Winston's *Adaptogens - Herbs for Strength, Stamina, and Stress Relief.*

Decoction

What you need:

- Medium size pot
- 2 teaspoons of dried schizandra berries
- 2 teaspoons of goji berries
- 2 teaspoons of hawthorn berries
- 16 oz / 500ml of water

1. Place all of the ingredients into the pot.
2. Bring to a simmer and allow to simmer for 20 to 30 minutes
3. Leave to steep for up to an hour.

Drink three cups a day, and aim for a morning, afternoon, and evening cup.

Tincture

I do get busy at certain periods and find I don't drink it daily, so I am also including the details on making the tincture of this natural healing remedy. The tincture is much easier to take three times a day, every day. Make the infusion in larger amounts, adjust the ingredients to match the amount of water, and try to consume daily until the tincture is ready. I do not like to blend this tincture.

What you need:

- 2 tablespoons of dried schizandra berries
- 2 tablespoons of goji berries
- 2 tablespoons of hawthorn berries
- Bottle of vodka or brandy (or red wine)

1. Fill a glass jar ⅓ full of an equal mix of hawthorn, goji, and schizandra berries.
2. Pour in your vodka or brandy (you can use red wine, too) and tighten the lid.
3. Shake daily and leave for 6 weeks or longer.

If you can't wait, pour some out to use after two weeks and let the rest sit. OR simply use the infusion daily until the tincture is ready.

This is a great remedy to help you be less stressed, have more energy, and support your heart, circulatory system, liver, kidneys, nervous system, adrenals, eyes, and brain. I have known many people with adrenal exhaustion for years to bounce back using this tincture and the nourishing herbal infusions daily. People have reported (over time) being able to reduce and even stop blood pressure medication with the guidance of their Doctor. Always work with your doctor if you are on medication.

Remedy 14 - Powerful Circulation Tonic

This powerful circulation tonic is great for improving circulation to the extremities. It has a positive effect on the heart and digestion.

What you need:

- Glass storage jar
- Pot
- 1 Slice of ginger rhizome 3 to 6 inches in size (peeled)
- 1 bottle of red wine or apple cider vinegar
- 1 teaspoon of cayenne pepper
- 3 sprigs of thyme
- 3 sprigs of rosemary

You can make this tonic in a number of ways:

Option 1:
1. Simply put the items in a glass
2. Pour in the wine or vinegar
3. Wait 6 weeks, shaking every day.

Option 2:
1. Pour the wine or vinegar into a blender
2. Add the ginger and cayenne pepper
3. Blend for 10 minutes and then strain back into the bottle or another glass jar
4. Add the rosemary and thyme. It can be used straight away but gets better as time goes on

Option 3:
1. Pour the wine or vinegar into a heat-resistant jar
2. Add ingredients to that jar.
3. Place the jar into a pan of water, bring to the boil and simmer for 10 minutes
4. Allow to cool completely before straining and storing in a glass jar/ bottle.

Take this at first in ½ teaspoon amounts and work up, but you should not need more than 1 teaspoon dose taken 2 to 3 times a day or every couple of hours if you need to.

All the options to make this tonic work well, but I prefer the last method. I enjoy the taste; I have also found that I can heat thyme and rosemary in a very dry red wine and take that in small glass amounts.

Remedy 15 - Circulation and Capillary Health

This remedy is great for tackling spider veins, varicose veins and more.

Tincture

What you need:

- Glass storage jar
- 100 grams of Hawthorn Berries
- 100 grams of Goji Berries
- 100 grams of Blueberries
- 1 Bottle of vodka or red wine

Vodka version

1. Simply put the items in a glass storage jar
2. Pour in the vodka
3. Wait 6 weeks, shaking every day.

Red wine version

1. Pour the wine into a heat-resistant jar
2. Add ingredients to that jar.
3. Place the jar into a pan of water, bring to the boil and simmer for 10 minutes

4. Allow to cool completely before straining and storing in a glass jar/
    bottle.

Whatever version you make, you can take 2ml (two droppers full) twice to four times daily.

I prefer the vodka version of this tincture. Let me know which one works best for you.

If you have circulation issues or problems with capillaries, spider veins, varicose veins, etc., then you should dose this multiple times per day. I find a tincture dropped into a warm glass of water or tea is easier than drinking the wine version.

I have known people to take this, plus daily herbal infusions and reverse spider veins and circulatory issues. This is also good for the tiny capillaries in the eyes.

Something else to consider if you suffer from poor circulation and capillary health would be to take a copper supplement and eat foods high in copper. People have found that eating citrus fruits with the pith (the white stuff on the outside of the soft fruit) and eating regular salads that include large amounts of watercress, beetroot, apples, olive, capers, and if you can eat it, buckwheat help. These are all high in rutin, which can protect the capillaries and improve circulation. You can juice or blend all of those foods together (except buckwheat), which I and others have done, but it doesn't taste as nice as eating them. These foods do work, and they have BIG health benefits beyond circulation.

Remedy 16 - Anxiety No More

Many people in the world right now are suffering from anxiety. From newspapers to news on TV, fear seems to be the currency of these media. No wonder anxiety and mental disorders are growing rapidly. There are many lifestyle things people can do to help combat anxiety, but two simple teas can help wonders. They both have a relaxing, anti-anxiety effect in people: jasmine and lemongrass tea + chamomile and passion flower can be drunk in combination during the day and before bed, respectively.

Simple to make, these two are GREAT tasting (makes a change) and work very well. I originally got this one from the guys at Neal's Yard. The original recipe had more herbs in it, but these combinations work. There is one for the daytime and one for the evening.

Day Time

What you need:

- Teapot
- 1 stem of Lemongrass
- 1 tablespoon Jasmine Flowers
- 200ml boiling water
- 100ml cold water
- A dash of lime if you desire

1. Chop the lemon grass and add to the teapot
2. Add the Jasmine flowers.
3. Pour 200 ml of boiling water into a measuring jug and add 100 ml of cold water
4. Pour into the teapot. Leave for 10 to 20 minutes and drink.

This makes two servings. It is as enjoyable cold as it is warm (in my opinion). Have it as your first morning tea and later in the morning to keep you feeling balanced. Add a dash of lime just before serving if you like. I prefer to add lime when it's cold; without lime when drunk warm.

Bed Time

What you need:

- Teapot
- 1 tbsp of chamomile flowers
- 2 tbsp of passion flower
- 300ml of boiled water

1. Place the flowers in a teapot
2. Pour over the boiled water (allow a boiled kettle to rest for a couple of minutes before pouring), then leave for 5 to 20 minutes.
3. Adjust to taste.

I have a large mug of this, so around 300ml to 350ml of water is enough for me. I leave it usually for 10 to 20 minutes, depending on what I go off to do while it brews!

This one can induce tiredness, which certainly does for me, so it's not ideal for daytime consumption. However, it helps me feel comfortably tired by bedtime if I drink a cup around an hour and a half before bed. For individuals with severe anxiety affecting their sleep, this remedy has proven effective in ushering them into dreamland in conjunction with daytime tea (consumed throughout the day).

Experiment with the dosage of each flower; the above works best for me and most people who use it, but feel free to adjust it. Always proceed cautiously when increasing the amounts.

I take the before-bed remedy with me on holiday and enjoy it nearly every night.

Down South - Bowel and Bladder

Remedy 17 - Spiced Apple Sauce

A straightforward remedy to help ease constipation and maintain regularity naturally and gently. While there may be situations where you need a more immediate solution, it's advisable to avoid relying on harsh laxatives regularly. This remedy, combined with sufficient hydration, can assist in restoring regular bowel movements. Below we have two ways of preparing this remedy, one raw, the other cooked.

Raw Applesauce

What you need to blend:

- 2 peeled and sliced up apples
- 1 tablespoon of cinnamon
- ½ teaspoon of clove
- 5 prunes
- 1 oz elderberries/blueberries and cranberry mix (or one of them)
- Touch of honey if needed.

1. Soak the dried fruit
2. Peel and chop the apples, place them into the blender, and cover with water.
3. Begin blending and add the spices and fruit, and continue blending

until the fruits and apples are thoroughly chopped and mixed.

Cooked Applesauce

Alternatively, you can use cooking apples and add them to a pan with a little water, cooking them down until almost soft. Add the fruits and spices when nearly cooked. Thoroughly mix or blend the ingredients when cooked (allow it to cool for a while before blending).

This mixture can be consumed by a spoonful or, as I prefer, mixed into yogurt to alleviate constipation and provide relief for stomach flu. It serves as a potent antioxidant and anti-parasitic remedy. If you're experiencing diarrhea, omit the prunes and possibly the dried fruit mix. Apples alone can help with diarrhea; however, I appreciate the added spices as they can act on any underlying cause of the issue.

This concoction can be delightful to consume, especially when warm in the winter, and is generally suitable for children. However, you might need to adjust the spice amounts, particularly for children.

Remedy 18 - Bladder Support - UTI Buster

This natural healing remedy again utilizes what you have in the kitchen cupboard. This bladder support - UTI buster first worked for my wife over a decade ago when she was suffering from a nasty urinary tract infection. You can start with half the dose below for the first day or two to get used to it or jump straight in. Do not use more than stated doses.

This is a two part remedy

What you need:

- ½ to 1 teaspoon of Bicarbonate of Soda
- ½ teaspoon of Cream of Tartar
- ½ teaspoon of a good whole food salt.
- Glass of warm water

1. ½ to 1 teaspoon of bicarbonate of soda in a glass of warm water. Take this first thing in the morning
2. ½ teaspoon of cream of tartar in a glass of warm water two times per day. Once in the afternoon, the second/last dose before bed. Also includes 1/4 tsp of a good whole food salt an hour before bed.

The aforementioned protocol, coupled with increased water intake and the inclusion of herbal teas such as thyme, rosemary, or yarrow throughout the day, can yield remarkable results. It's advisable to cut out sugar until the infection is completely resolved.

For individuals dealing with chronic recurring urinary tract infections, maintaining a consistent intake of fluids along with pure cranberry juice containing added D-mannose can be a lifesaver. I once knew a man grappling with several chronic health issues and decades of recurrent UTIs who adopted the natural healing remedy mentioned above, incorporating herbal teas and cranberry juice. Not only did he cease experiencing chronic UTIs, but his other health conditions also became more manageable.

NOTE: Although I have seen this natural healing remedy work miracles and work where antibiotics had failed, UTIs can cause serious health issues, especially if they become acute and affect the kidneys, so please always seek medical advice.

Caution - If you are on medication or have kidney issues, please check with your medical practitioner before trying this natural healing remedy. Also, do not go above stated doses. Cream of tartar contains high potassium levels, an essential element for our bodies that many people do not get enough of. BUT the body has a small tolerance window for potassium compared to sodium.

Where It All Began For Me

<u>Remedy 19 - My Amazing Gout Creation – Gout-be-Gone</u>

This is the natural healing remedy that set me on the path to study. As mentioned earlier, I began experiencing severe gout attacks at a young age. People were skeptical when gout first manifested around the age of 23 or 24. I would endure two to three attacks annually, necessitating the use of potent medications, such as indomethacin, to alleviate the pain and inflammation. Each time, I found myself on these medications for weeks to months. The pain was so intense that even putting on a sock became unbearable.

Following the acute phase, I had to wear soft black shoes instead of my usual smart 'dress' shoes to work, as any other footwear would cause discomfort for several weeks post-attack. I had to adopt peculiar half steps, walking very slowly, whereas I usually walked at an accelerated pace. Upon disembarking from the underground tube in London, I would patiently wait for the crowd to pass before slowly making my way out of the station, feeling like a decrepit old man.

To cut a long story short, I stumbled upon Tony Pantalleresco on YouTube one day. He suggested a natural remedy that I thought might work. Since the shop didn't have papaya, I substituted it with pineapple, known for its enzyme content that breaks down proteins and has anti-inflammatory properties. I concocted this natural healing remedy and waited a full week. One Saturday night, I was going out with my girlfriend (now wife) to a friend's 30th birthday party. I insisted on taking a taxi, and I swore off alcohol because the gout was flaring up.

A few hours before heading out, I consumed the remainder of the natural healing remedy, probably three or four doses, along with four serrapeptase enzymes. I swallowed it down, hoping I wouldn't have to limp during the evening. After some time, I can't recall precisely—between 30 and 60 minutes, I believe—I felt diminished pain. Then, a fizzing sensation occurred in my swollen toe. It persisted for a while until, suddenly, the pain vanished. The swelling disappeared. It was normal!

Typically, gout would linger, but with this natural healing remedy, it vanished completely. We canceled the taxi and walked to the party. I was ecstatic, running up and down the road, exclaiming that the pain was gone. I indulged in multiple pints of beer that night (for science), and nothing happened. Since then, approximately 15 years ago, I've experienced a few twinges, usually triggered by excessive consumption of beans/pulses or dehydration. The only time I took medication in the last 15 years was during a holiday in Zante, Greece. After a few days of insufficient water intake, a bit of pain set in. I purchased tablets from the local chemist for that day and the next, and that was it. For me, it served as a warning rather than a genuine gout attack. Contrary to what the doctor told me years ago, protein doesn't seem to affect me. Black beans and dehydration do, along with excessive consumption of shrimp and liver. However, considering the severity of my gout in my twenties, I can confidently say that I am now living gout-free. This remedy has also proven effective for friends dealing with gout, arthritic hands, and painful knees.

Gout-Be-Gone

What you need:

- Glass container with airtight lid
- 1 fresh Pineapple,
- 2 tablespoons of cinnamon powder
- 1 tablespoon of Ginger powder
- 2 tablespoons of Turmeric powder
- Aloe Vera Juice.
- If you wish to supercharge this, then some systemic enzymes

1. Peel and then cut the pineapple up into chunks
2. Put in a glass container and add:
3. 2 tablespoons of Turmeric powder
4. 2 tablespoons of Cinnamon powder
5. 1 tablespoon of Ginger Powder
6. Mix it up and cover all of the pineapple in the powders.
7. Put the lid on and leave for a week.
8. After 1 week, put it in a blender and add enough Aloe Vera Juice to cover and allow you to blend it.
9. Filter the bits out. Use one ounce at a time 3 to 4 times a day.

If you can buy supplements, take some systemic enzymes when you take the natural healing remedy. This will help supercharge the results.

Alternatives :

Use papaya instead of pineapple, or use both.

Use fresh ginger juice instead of ginger powder when you add the aloe vera juice. Ginger juice is loaded with enzymes.

Want it NOW? - Do the above so you have one fermenting, but also use another pineapple. This time, juice or blend the pineapple right away, add the turmeric and cinnamon powders, cut them down to just 1 tablespoon and then use fresh ginger juice and aloe vera juice.

Let me know how it works for you. I hope it works as well as it did for me all those years ago. My brother told me that when his wife was giving birth to their first child, the female nurse told him that gout (he was having an attack – not great timing!) was the most pain a man could feel and was worse than the pain of childbirth! It didn't go down too well with his wife.

If you experience success with any of the 19 natural healing remedies in this book, please let us know by contacting 19remediesthatwork@ gmail.com with "Testimonial" in the subject line. We value hearing all the details, and if you observe any improvements, please share them. Your feedback is greatly appreciated.

Section 4

Play with the 19 natural healing remedies

Here you have it: the 19 natural healing remedies that work. All 19 are easy to make, cheaply, effective, and have no terrible side effects. While some of you may be familiar with a few of these natural healing remedies, others may be new to you.

Now, your next step is to choose one to try and see if it can contribute to your journey towards improved health. Whether you pick one that others have found effective for similar issues or opt for one with ingredients readily available at home, the key is to get involved and start creating that natural healing remedy.

In addition to the specific ingredients outlined for each of the 19 natural healing remedies, I've also provided alternatives. The goal is to emphasize that although these remedies are potent and effective, they are not like a laboratory science experiment where a slight error could lead to an explosion. We're not baking a cake, so the measurements don't need to be exact. Feel free to play with the ingredients, figure out what your body tolerates best, and don't hesitate to experiment. For instance, powdered ginger can be a suitable substitute if fresh ginger is unavailable for your honey and ginger remedy.

One common pitfall that has been significant in my life is the tendency to postpone tasks if they can't be done perfectly. However, as we all know, 'later' often never comes. So, just do it! Enjoy the process, have fun, and reap the benefits.

I've included profiles of all the ingredients, detailing their benefits and traditional uses. This information empowers you to use your imagination and create your own combinations. It might result in concoctions that taste terrible or are too spicy, but that's all part of the learning process. You might also discover that while one of the 19 natural healing remedies works well for you, it doesn't provide a 100% resolution. In that case, tweak it! Many people have done so over the years, often due to the taste of certain remedies.

If just one or a few of the 19 natural healing remedies help eliminate a health issue completely, that's amazing! This is why I felt the need to share these remedies beyond my circle of friends and family. Some have reported reducing their prescription drugs and being content with that change. Others have continued their journeys and successfully stopped all medication, expressing amazement and gratitude. However, as you may have realized, I prefer comprehensive solutions.

Achieving that may require a bit of extra effort—playing with the remedies to tailor them to your individual needs or using them more regularly, even combining several or all of them. You'll need to find the right balance of effort and convenience for the results you're satisfied with. I genuinely hope that every person trying these 19 natural healing remedies finds at least one that works miracles, as they have for myself, friends, and family.

As I write this, I'm reminded that I haven't made many of the 19 natural healing remedies for a while. This is both a positive and a not-so-good thing. On one hand, people tend to think of 'remedies' as something to take when sick, and that's the true meaning of the word. However, some of the remedies here would be beneficial to incorporate into our lives regularly as a preventative measure. For example, the natural healing remedy – Gout-be-Gone, which I used to overcome debilitating gout, would be ideal to take for a week or so several times a year to provide the body with an anti-inflammatory, digestion-enhancing, circulation-improving boost. It serves as a timely reminder that we should all be integrating these 19 natural healing remedies into our daily lives.

While I've emphasized that these remedies are safe, exercise caution and remember to consult your medical practitioner when necessary. Each person is unique, and you may have a higher or lower tolerance to the ingredients used in these natural healing remedies.

Section 5

Real-life examples of the 19 natural healing remedies In action!

Gout

This is where my journey truly began. I had an interest in nutrition before my first gout attack, primarily for fat loss and muscle gain. My studies and experimentation with nutrition provided invaluable insights into how commonly held beliefs can be misleading.

Every day, we encounter news articles, mainstream TV adverts, and even medical professionals repeating the same, often inaccurate, nutrition advice as if it were fact. In my opinion, for the best advice on getting in shape, consulting a bodybuilder is often more beneficial. While being in shape and healthy don't always align, shedding excess fat often significantly improves overall health, regardless of the diet or fad one might follow.

I discovered that once your mind is exposed to the realization that widely accepted information is often wrong, it becomes challenging to accept anything at face value. This skepticism became ingrained in my thinking.

Due to my interest in weightlifting and diets, I started listening to podcasts on health, a relatively new trend at the time. I delved into books on vitamins, minerals, and their role in human biochemistry. The information was eye-opening. I experimented with fasting, juicing, and high-dose vitamin therapies, yielding positive results. However, despite these positive changes, I was still a young man working a job I didn't particularly enjoy in London, eagerly awaiting the weekends. The weekends, which often stretched from Thursday to Monday, became the focal point of my life, depending on my financial situation.

Yes, I know; we live, and we learn.

At the age of 23, I embarked on driving lessons amidst experiencing severe bouts of gout. These attacks typically began overnight and were excruciatingly painful. My big toe joint would redden, swell, and throb with pain, making it intolerable even for a bed sheet or sock. I endured numerous gout episodes over the years, necessitating powerful painkillers. Even after the worst had passed, the pain lingered, requiring weeks of continued medication just to make it to work. I recall having to purchase soft black shoes for the days when my regular smart work shoes proved too painful. I would cautiously make my way to the station, clad in my special soft shoes, avoiding crowded tubes, fearing someone stepping on my foot. Getting off the tube required waiting for the majority to pass before attempting a slow exit, reminiscent of a gout-induced hobble. Not an ideal situation in your early and mid-twenties.

These episodes would persist for many weeks, sometimes up to three months, occurring two to three times a year. Consequently, I spent a significant portion of the year in pain from gout. Even with more mobility in my soft shoes, walking remained painful. I acknowledge that my own choices prolonged these bouts of gout. Many times, I popped painkillers before heading out to pubs or bars, exacerbating the issue. If only I had learned early what triggered my gout and made the necessary lifestyle changes, I might not have suffered for so long.

As mentioned earlier, I consulted a doctor who recommended high doses of medication for the rest of my life. While I have criticized doctors for their prescription-focused approach, I understand the reasons behind it. Many individuals prefer maintaining their existing lifestyle, even if it leads to illness, relying on medication to manage the consequences. When the medication's effectiveness wanes or causes additional issues, some resign themselves to the situation, believing there's nothing more to be done.

A striking example is my sister's encounter with a patient in a local hospital. The man had severe gout in almost every joint, making him exceptionally miserable. His gout was primarily caused by his relentless consumption of liver, a food he loved. Liver featured in every meal— liver pate sandwiches, liver for lunch, and liver for dinner. Despite being aware of the health risks, he refused to stop. While an extreme case, it illustrates a common human tendency. Many of us engage in activities we know are detrimental simply because we enjoy them and are resistant to change. However, I believe everyone has a turning point.

For me, the prospect of being on medication for life was my turning point. I'm uncertain why the severe gout attacks in my early twenties didn't prompt an earlier realization that I needed to change. I persisted in drinking, relying on strong pain medications, and limping around. Fortunately, my stubbornness outweighed my laziness, and I wasn't content with the doctor's prescription for lifelong medication. I resolved to find my own way out of gout.

I began reading and discovered that certain foods aggravated gout, different from the ones my doctor had listed. For me, lentils and beans, especially black beans, trigger a 'twinge' if consumed twice a week. I can enjoy liver weekly but not more frequently. As someone who had dealt with gut issues throughout my life, and considering the correlation between gut problems and gout, I started adjusting my diet.

Nevertheless, gout continued to resurface intermittently, prompting me to persist in my search for a solution. That's when I stumbled upon Tony Pantalereco on YouTube. His videos, blending foods and herbs in ways I had never seen before, were a revelation. Unlike the courses and books I had previously explored, Tony's approach incorporated herbs and foods uniquely. I reached out to him regarding my gout, seeking any advice he could offer. Tony was incredibly helpful and directed me to his video on fermented papaya. Despite not finding papaya, I opted for pineapple and embarked on creating the recipe for Natural Health Remedy number 19 in this book.

After a week of fermenting the ingredients as Tony recommended, I began using the remedy alongside systemic enzymes. A few days into the treatment, I found myself still relying on painkillers for the latest gout episode. It was the weekend, and I was with my girlfriend at my flat in Essex, preparing to attend her friend's 30th birthday party. I was in the midst of a gout attack, making it painful, but with soft shoes, I could manage. We planned to book a taxi as the venue was a bit far for me to hobble, walking on the heel of my foot, trying to avoid putting pressure on my big toe.

By this time, I had learned the importance of staying hydrated and avoiding alcohol (at least until the pain subsided). The plan was set: wear soft shoes, take a taxi, drink plenty of water, and abstain from alcohol. All of this at a party with people I didn't know. It presented quite a challenge!

Having taken my Gout-be-Gone remedy for a few days in small amounts multiple times a day, I neared the end of the concoction. A couple of hours before leaving for the party, I consumed the remaining portion (around 4 ounces) along with a handful of systemic enzymes. I drank a considerable amount of water with the enzymes. Somewhere between 30 to 60 minutes later, a strange sensation enveloped my big toe. It was fizzing, and after a few minutes, my toe joint began to reduce swelling, allowing me to move my toe. The pain was fading, feeling almost miraculous. As we prepared to leave, the plan changed. No taxi was needed. I still put on my soft shoes (just in case), but I walked 20 to 30 minutes to the venue. In fact, I was running up and down the street, exclaiming to my girlfriend, "Look, no pain" – a bit like a madman. Anyone who has suffered gout knows this doesn't happen. I was astonished.

Regrettably, as a young man who still enjoyed the occasional drink on nights out, I decided to put my newfound remedy to the test. Not only did we walk to and from the venue, but I also drank some water and wine. No gout! The next morning, still no gout! My mind was blown. I had 'cured' my gout.

That was around 16 years ago. Since that transformative night, I haven't experienced a full-blown gout attack. I've had the occasional 'twinge' if I consumed liver two days in a row, let myself get dehydrated, or ate black beans, but never a full-on gout attack.

This positive outcome propelled me into a journey of further discovery, and I've learned an incredible amount. I've encountered remarkable individuals who have successfully reversed almost every type of disease over the years. Once you realise such transformations are possible, you start looking at the world differently. Strangely, this realization can be overwhelming for some people. They resist seeing life differently, avoiding having their beliefs challenged or their minds blown. It's undoubtedly a challenging shift, especially when surrounded by like-minded individuals. Nevertheless, I urge you to take the leap and test what is and isn't possible for yourself, on yourself, first.

I must emphasize that while I still consider my Gout-be-Gone a cure—a miracle of my own—there are practices I continue to this day to ward off any potential flare-ups. Below is a list of everything I do:

1) **Stay Hydrated**: Drink plenty of water and herbal infusions, tea, or fresh juice daily. Adequate hydration is crucial and often underestimated. Regularly use the toilet to ensure proper urination.

2) **Identify Trigger Foods**: Determine which foods tend to cause flare-ups for you. While there are general recommendations for individuals prone to gout, it is a highly individual matter. While I don't completely avoid potential trigger foods, I don't consume them excessively, either.

3) **Systemic Enzymes**: Consider using systemic enzymes if feasible. After the age of 27, there's an argument for everyone to take enzymes to support overall health. Enzymes play a role in breaking down foreign proteins, improving circulation, aiding liver detoxification, reducing scar tissue and inflammation, and enhancing digestion.

4) **Incorporate Anti-Inflammatory Foods**: Consume anti-inflammatory foods daily, particularly those rich in protein-digesting enzymes such as pineapple, papaya, kiwi, and ginger. Whether eaten, juiced or in other

forms, ensure they are part of your regular diet.

5) **Prevent Constipation**: Avoid constipation, as gout attacks have been observed to occur after episodes of constipation. Constipation is often linked to dehydration, causing stress on the body and hindering detoxification processes.

These practices require minimal effort but can significantly contribute to gout management. Identifying specific trigger foods is crucial. In my case, prune juice, black beans, and lentils trigger gout, which was not initially on the list provided by the doctor. While the doctor recommended limiting animal protein and encouraging beans and lentils, I found I could consume ample animal protein without issue. Understanding your primary triggers is essential.

Hydration is paramount and can provide some leeway when consuming alcohol or trigger foods. The herbal infusions in this book, along with Natural Healing Remedy number 19, have played a key role in helping me live gout and drug-free.

I've encountered numerous individuals with gout success stories similar to mine, and many have experienced varying degrees of improvement. For some, gout symptoms gradually diminish and stay away. In contrast, others may have occasional relapses but not as severe or prolonged. Those who identify trigger foods, avoid them, and maintain good hydration seem to bid farewell to gout after using Natural Healing Remedy number 19. Some use it periodically or in modified forms when consuming trigger foods. Those who struggle with maintaining hydration or consistently avoiding trigger foods may not fare as well. But they still appreciate the positive impact of the 19 natural healing remedies on their gout outcomes. This, in my view, speaks volumes about the effectiveness of these approaches.

Joint Pain

I experienced significant knee pain during my weightlifting sessions. Although I initially relied on supplements to address joint pain, the cost and certain high doses of vitamins in the products prompted me to explore a natural alternative.

Upon hearing on a radio show that plain gelatine had been studied for its potential incorporation into joints if taken 30 minutes before a workout, I decided to give it a try. Surprisingly, I decided to create a bone and joint remedy along with a reduction in pain and inflammation in my knee joints.

I already incorporated nourishing herbal infusions, following the approach popularized by herbalist Susan Weed, though not as consistently as I should have. I resumed daily intake of these infusions and created a mixed infusion using nettle leaf, oatstraw, and horsetail. To this mix, I added gelatine to create a jelly, either dissolving it while hot or letting it bloom and then blending the entire mixture. Within a week, I noticed positive effects on my joint pain. Still feeling the need for more sulfur, I developed the Sulfur Super Power Soup.

Regular consumption of this combination completely alleviated my knee pain, and even lingering shoulder pain disappeared. After sharing these remedies with weightlifting friends, they, too, incorporated the drink daily and had the soup as needed or if pain recurred. I witnessed individuals with shoulder, hip, lower back, and knee pain experience symptom relief with consistent use of these Natural Healing Remedies.

The potential side effects include increased energy, more flexible arteries, a calmed nervous system, improved hair and nail growth, and healthier kidneys and liver. Frequent consumption of the soup has even shown improvements in liver function, as evidenced by enzyme tests.

Constipation Gone

I understand the frustrations associated with constipation, as I have personally struggled with gut and bowel issues from a young age. My earliest memory of a potential gastrointestinal issue involves accidentally swallowing a metal bolt when I was around 4 or 5 years old. Despite thorough examinations, including X-rays, the bolt was never found and was assumed to have passed through naturally.

Another contributor to my gut issues was gluten intolerance, a condition I discovered later in life. Consuming gluten-rich foods, particularly bread, exacerbated my symptoms. Despite seeking medical advice and being diagnosed with irritable bowel syndrome (IBS), the provided food list did not align with my individual needs. Only after reading Robb Wolf's book, *The Paleo Diet*, did I learn about the detrimental effects of gluten on the gut and overall health. Eliminating gluten from my diet significantly improved my gut health despite my initial reluctance to give up beloved gluten-containing foods.

This experience underscores the importance of identifying the root cause of constipation. Factors such as food intolerances, dehydration, magnesium deficiency, and inadequate soluble fiber intake can contribute to bowel issues. While the natural healing remedy for constipation outlined in this book is effective, understanding and addressing the underlying cause is crucial.

For individuals experiencing severe constipation, defined by infrequent bowel movements (a couple of times per week), hydration plays a pivotal role. Consuming nourishing herbal infusions, such as the one described in natural healing remedy number 1, is recommended. Adding a crystal of high-quality Celtic Sea salt to the tongue before drinking the infusion aids in hydration. Additionally, juicing a combination of cucumber, celery, carrot, and apple or blending them into a smoothie helps maintain proper hydration and provides essential nutrients for optimal bowel function.

Hydration alone can address various health issues and ensure the necessary nutrients for proper bowel function. The Spiced Apple Sauce highlighted in this book has proven effective for individuals with infrequent bowel movements. This advice is particularly relevant for individuals aged 60 and above, as proper hydration becomes even more critical, especially in settings like hospitals or care homes where older individuals may not drink enough fluids.

TIP - Don't guzzle your drinks.

I got into the habit of drinking fast! I used to start the night by drinking 5 pints in the first hour when I went out. I don't know why; I just always drank fast. Water at home, I would guzzle a pint in seconds. I was drinking many liters of water when I was told on more than one occasion that I showed signs of dehydration. I went for a blood draw one day, and the nurse said, "You are dehydrated." I replied, "No way. I drink liters of water daily." She said, "Maybe you drink too much." I thought she was talking nonsense.

I also did a 24-hour urine test years ago. I recorded the amount peed at over 5 liters. The lab called a few days later from the United States to ask if I had written the volume down correctly. It turns out drinking lots of water doesn't mean you get properly hydrated! You need to sip your fluids and minerals to help to hydrate you.

Spiced Apple Sauce

The recipe for this is versatile. You can use it cold and blended if you are in a hurry, on a warm summer day, or heated in a pan for a winter treat. Use prunes if constipated; remove them to help ease diarrhea. This one was born out of one from Tony Pantalleresco.

I used this to good effect, so I passed this on for the first time to a friend who was having issues while working abroad in Spain. It was summer; the weather was hot, the food was different, and his job put a lot of stress on him. He was using the toilet every other day with a struggle if he was lucky and often using drugs to help him go. We had a discussion and identified several things:

1. He wasn't drinking enough, and when he did drink, it was when he was very thirsty and would drink a bottle of water in one go. He also drank a pint of ice-cold water with his evening meal.
2. His job meant he was very stressed, and work talk was constant, even at night when he had dinner.
3. He was eating like he was on holiday and had too many stodgy foods for breakfast, lunch, and dinner.
4. He was drinking two glasses of wine with his evening meal alongside the pint of ice-cold water.

He had been out there for three months and lived how most people live on a one-week holiday. We identified the issues above; not much detective work went into it, really; these things are obvious when you know what to look for. Based on these 4 points, he made the following changes:

1. He didn't want to do infusions, but he bought Celtic Sea salt, put one large or two small crystals on his tongue, and drank them down first thing in the morning before anything else, then again 60 to 30 minutes pre-lunch, and the same for dinner. He also made a two-liter bottle of water each day with mint and cucumber in it and sipped on that throughout the day.

2. If work talk over dinner was unavoidable, he would try to cut it off and relax before the end of the meal and spend more time actively relaxing before bed.

3. He was unwilling to change his food much, but he found he wasn't eating so much when drinking a glass of water pre-meals.

4. He stopped drinking wine some nights, and he reduced his consumption to only one glass other nights. He wouldn't stop, so the deal was that the glass of water he drank with salt before his evening meal would be 1 pint, starting an hour before the meal and finishing no later than 20 minutes before his meal. The pint of iced water with his meal was gone. We replaced it with a small glass of room temperature water with lemon sipped slowly, somewhere between an hour post-meal and bedtime. He would also drink a pint of cucumber and mint water or water with a crystal of Celtic salt.

5. He made the Spiced Apple Sauce and took a three-tablespoon dose at a time. He took this after his water in the morning but before breakfast and again before bed, whatever time was comfortable for him.

As it turned out, he made the Spiced Apple Sauce cold in his blender most of the time and added more water so he could drink it down. He got to enjoy the spicy taste, and even more so the effects and would sometimes take it during the day, too. Originally, I said to take it four times a day as his constipation was bad, but at the time, he could only manage two times a day. That dose, along with the additional hydration and small changes we made, was a winner. After a couple of days, he was very happy. After around ten days, he dropped the prunes to two, and then a week or so later, he started to leave them out and add them when he felt like it or felt he might need them. That was his intuition talking to him. Prunes are great but, in a way, are a little forceful on the bowel, and I prefer not to be reliant on them. Apples are a perfect food to balance the bowel. That said, like myself and many others, he now takes it here and there, not daily, and he is a very happy man.

He, like others, tells me that it feels like a weight has been lifted when they get over chronic constipation. There are still so many people suffering from this. This will not only lead to a lifetime of stress and discomfort but, eventually, other health problems.

A side effect is that people report a happy feeling when constipation is lifted; they are less angry, have more energy and enjoy life more. Also, people tend to see gut issues disappear or become greatly reduced. On two occasions, my friend was the only person who ate out in a restaurant and didn't get sick. He believes now that (as many report back) he gets colds and flus less often. This is the power of food and spices.

The same guy passed the Spiced Apple Sauce remedy on to his father, who was in an assisted living facility. He was 85 and not doing too well. Increasing his hydration was difficult, but it was done to a degree. His father didn't like the spice, so that was left out at first. He was on many medications which bunged him up, and so he was put on laxatives. I have seen this over and over within my own family. They are given multiple drugs; a side effect of all of these is constipation, so they are also prescribed laxatives. There is often no plan in place to come off, reduce or get past the use of all the medication, meaning you are left on the laxatives. In older people, this can mean they end up in a real mess. It's a horrible vicious circle.

The result was his father, who was struggling to go to the toilet twice a week, got back to being regular. No urgency, just morality, and he was very happy. His father enjoys the Spiced Apple Sauce warm with yogurt for breakfast some mornings or, like his son, as a drink, taken as a shot during the day. Even better, I have been told that staff and other residents in the assisted living facility also use this remedy. That is what natural healing remedies are about.

As you have just read, I gave a friend a natural healing remedy but didn't just say, "Take this. If you do, it will work." For many people, they haven't changed anything else; they just took the natural healing remedy and had good results. However, in the long term, we need to consider why the issue is happening and make small, simple adjustments to truly improve our health.

Indigestion/ Acid Reflux

Acid reflux is a significant issue, ranging from a mild inconvenience to a highly painful and potentially problematic condition for long-term health. The prevailing belief about acid reflux is that excessive stomach acid production is the culprit, leading individuals to take medications to neutralize the acid. While effective in the short term, the focus on immediate relief raises concerns about the potential long-term consequences.

Practitioners adopting a more holistic or natural approach view indigestion as more of a problem related to insufficient stomach acid. This perspective considers the individual nature of this issue. The rationale behind this approach is that a lack of stomach acid can result in inadequate or delayed digestion of food in the gut, leading to fermentation and acid buildup. People often resort to medications to alleviate acid reflux, preventing it from moving back up into the esophagus. However, this strategy can create additional problems as proper acid levels are essential, especially for breaking down proteins. Research suggests a correlation between regular use of antacid medications and various long-term health issues.

Natural healing remedy number 10 focuses on ensuring optimal stomach function by maintaining appropriate levels of stomach acid. This approach aids in the proper digestion of incoming food, facilitating the breakdown of foods and their timely passage into the small intestine.

Customer cures severe acid reflux

I used to own an online supplement store where I sold a variety of health supplements. Customers often posed challenging questions about products, and responding was tricky due to restrictions on making suggestions or offering advice as a supplement store owner. Despite decades of clinical use and studies supporting many supplements, extreme caution was necessary in communication. Typically, my responses were confined to statements like, "This product supports the structure and function of the body."

One day, a customer emailed seeking a solution for severe acid reflux that OTC drugs could no longer alleviate. Having witnessed the effectiveness of natural healing remedy number 9 - Acid Reflux Emergency Formula on numerous occasions, I recommended it. The customer was surprised that I didn't attempt to sell him something. I clarified that it was an inexpensive, easy, and effective formula. However, I emphasized the need to use it with cream of tartar due to its high potassium content, specifying its application for emergencies to halt the burning sensation. I also provided links for purchasing herbal bitters and shared Natural Healing Remedy number 10 - Indigestion / Acid Reflux Remedy. After expressing gratitude, I heard nothing further, a common occurrence, particularly with individuals less health-conscious who seek supplements or herbs as they would conventional drugs. It's frustrating, yet understandable, as medication simplifies life.

Several months later, I received another email from the same customer. He had followed my advice, utilized the suggested natural healing remedies, and acquired herbal bitters. Delighted with the outcomes, he had ceased medication entirely, rarely requiring the Acid Reflux Emergency Formula. He had developed an affinity for natural healing remedy number 10, incorporating it into his routine as a tea. According to him, his digestion had improved by 100%, eliminating bloating, fullness, gas, and acid reflux burning in his esophagus. While occasionally taking bicarbonate of soda in water in the morning and a small amount of cream of tartar before bed for other health reasons, he no longer experienced digestive issues.

I firmly believe in the importance of herbal bitters. With their historical presence in our diets, they induce a bitter taste that stimulates saliva and initiates stomach acid production. This prepares the pancreas for bile production and signals the entire digestive tract for overall readiness. Besides the absence of bitter foods in modern diets, the increased sugar consumption puts stress on organs. Bitters can play a crucial role in reducing blood sugar levels and mitigating the associated damage.

A Tea or Two For a World of Anxiety

Personally, I've always adopted a mindset of not caring too much, sometimes to an extreme extent, leading to considerable abuse of my body in my younger years. While maintaining a healthy level of concern and connection with the world is essential, the information overload we face today is overwhelming. My wife, in particular, experiences anxiety due to this incessant barrage of information. Instead of impartially reporting news, the media seems inclined towards negative commentaries and the promotion of fear. Although we generally avoid watching the news, a recent exposure to the 10 pm news highlighted the pervasive use of the word 'crisis' nine times in two and a half minutes! We are inundated not only with local and interesting international news but also with distressing global events. While empathetic, I believe that constant exposure to bad, shocking, disgusting, and scary news before bedtime is detrimental to mental well-being. I am not suggesting a lack of empathy. Rather, I question the necessity of subjecting our brains to an excess of distressing information in a 24-hour period. The resulting anxiety is a significant concern, and it would be refreshing if news segments concluded with something positive, optimistic, and uplifting.

My wife and I perceive a pandemic of anxiety affecting people of all ages. Lifestyle choices, dietary considerations, and supplements can contribute to anxiety reduction. I have witnessed the efficacy of natural healing remedy number 16 – Anxiety No More repeatedly. What's more, it even tastes good!

The first time I brewed the Anxiety No More tea myself was during a holiday. Wanting to enjoy the sun and relax while ensuring a good night's sleep without resorting to my usual holiday drink, wine, I visited a local health shop. I purchased Chamomile and Passionflower in dried herb form, steeping them in boiling water. The results were excellent, aiding in a restful night's sleep without the need for alcohol, which significantly impacts sleep quality.

I have recommended this Natural Healing Remedy to numerous individuals. While it constitutes a classic combination that works well in the evenings, many people seek something non-sedating for daytime use. Consulting a book by Neal's Yard, I identified a mix of herbs that contained too many ingredients for ease of use. I created a daytime tea by simplifying it to just lemongrass and jasmine flowers. In ample amounts, these ingredients effectively alleviate anxiety, induce relaxation, and, remarkably, bring smiles to people's faces.

One notable instance involved a friend who had benefited from other remedies. She approached me about a friend of hers struggling with heightened anxiety after quitting smoking. While powerful herbs exist for treating anxiety, lacking a detailed consultation with the lady, I recommended a rotation of nourishing herbal infusions—Oatstraw, Nettle, Oatstraw, Hawthorn, Oatstraw, Linden, Oatstraw. Additionally, I suggested the Lemongrass and Jasmine Flower tea in the morning, late morning, and before dinner. For the evening, I recommended chamomile and passionflower bedtime tea.

Since she was a friend of a friend, I sent her 500g of each herb in dried form on the condition that she would use them and report back after a month. After ten days, my friend informed me that the lady found the herbal infusions to make her excessively tired during the day, disrupting her usual routine. While she felt more relaxed in the evening and experienced improved sleep, her mind remained active with myriad thoughts before falling asleep.

Reflecting on this, I considered whether the lady's body was reacting adversely due to nutrient influx or if the infusions were too potent. Typically, people starting herbal infusions felt energized, but in this case, it seemed otherwise. Following the principle of "when you hear the sound of hoofs, first think horses before you think Zebra," I asked my friend to confirm the lady's exact intake. The issue became apparent—she was preparing the nourishing herbal infusions as tea (one teaspoon to a cup of water, brewed for five minutes) instead of the recommended method (1 oz in one liter of water, left to brew overnight). However, the primary mistake was switching the teas. She was consuming chamomile and passionflower bedtime tea during the day and lemongrass and jasmine flower daytime tea an hour before bed.

I clarified the confusion, and within four to five weeks, my friend informed me that the lady wanted to express her gratitude, pay me for the herbs, and obtain information on purchasing them in bulk. Her sleep had improved, and she woke up feeling refreshed and relaxed. Anxiety was virtually non-existent unless dealing with a serious issue. She had quit her five cups of daily coffee, as well as smoking, preferring herbal infusions and teas. She felt more focused and clear-headed, even resuming activities such as painting and dating, which she hadn't done in over twenty years. Last I heard, she was considering studying herbalism.

So, there you have it. I could continue sharing numerous real-life situations where these 19 natural healing remedies have genuinely helped people. Instead of providing an extensive list, I wanted to delve into a few detailed instances to illustrate why and how individuals have successfully used them.

I firmly believe that everyone should incorporate these 19 natural herbal remedies into their daily routine. This approach provides a solid foundation for supporting every cell, organ, and system in the body. Remedies for coughs can be prepared in early autumn as a precaution for winter, and those for circulation should be considered as we age or if our physical activity decreases. Integrating Natural Healing Remedies can be an enjoyable way to enhance life quality, not just for minor issues like coughs, colds, constipation, and indigestion but also for more serious diseases that are on the rise.

I genuinely hope you find these 19 natural healing remedies as beneficial as my friends and family have, with some experiencing dramatic, life-changing results. I encourage you to use, adapt, and share these remedies. If you have your own versions or success stories, please share them with me at 19remediesthatwork@gmail.com with "Testimonial" in the title.

I am living proof that incredible things can happen when you maintain an open mind, determination, perhaps a bit of stubbornness, and a willingness to try new things. I often reminisce about the day I felt that fizz in my toe and witnessed my painful gout vanish for good. Months of agony, specialized shoes, difficulty walking, and potent medications simply disappeared because I discovered the modern-day alchemist Tony Pantalleresco and dared to try his unconventional remedy.

In closing, I want to express my gratitude for reading. I strongly encourage you to implement these 19 natural healing remedies now. Be healthy, and ignore those who say you can't because I promise you you can. Think outside the box, don't succumb to dogma, move forward, and TAKE BACK YOUR HEALTH.

If you experience success with any of the 19 natural healing remedies in this book, please share your story with me at 19remediesthatwork@gmail.com using "Testimonial" in the title. We love hearing all the details, and if you make improvements, please do share them.

Section 6

Resources

Tony Pantallaresco - Herbalist alchemist. Tony describes himself as just a guy who knows some stuff. I learned a lot about natural remedies and started experimenting with herbs because of Tony. He has a website in Canada, loads of free material on his website and YouTube, and sells bespoke remedies. Check him out at http://augmentinforce.50webs.com/

Susan Weed - Susan is a well-known herbalist, Green Goddess, and promotes herbalism, 'The Wise Woman Way.' Susan popularized nourishing herbal infusions, has a radio show, and many books on herbs, healing, and women's health at http://www.herbshealing.com/

David Winston - A herbalist for over 40, maybe 50 years, David has a huge amount of clinical experience and is trained in several herbal healing modalities. David has a unique knowledge of ancient herbal wisdom and the latest scientific research. Check out David's products at https://www.herbalist-alchemist.com/

Neals Yard - https://www.nealsyardremedies.com/

Guedo Mase – A great herbalist who tells a story like no one else. https://www.simonandschuster.com/authors/Guido-Mase/410052592

Pubmed - https://pubmed.ncbi.nlm.nih.gov/

D. C Jarvis - https://www.amazon.co.uk/MEDICINE-cider-vinegar-health-Doctors-secrets/dp/B00XLOEWDS

Dr Mark Sircus - https://www.everand.com/author/417012681/Dr-Mark-Sircus

Dr Jerry Tennant - https://tennantinstitute.com/

Dr John Christopher - https://www.herballegacy.com/

Dr Wong - An amazing traditional Naturopath, Dr Wong has a wide range of knowledge, he is a PHD, a martial Arts hall of famer, he has been practicing natural medicine for 45 years, Dr Wong is a world leading expert on Systemic enzymes, and so much more. I don't have the room here to share a small fraction of his achievements. For THE best Enzymes and other products in the world, visit https://drwongsessentials.com/ If you are in Europe or the UK you can purchase direct from the US or email us at 19remediesthatwork@gmail.com and we will get you the best current place to purchase Dr Wong's products in Europe and the UK.

Gerson Therapy - https://gerson.org/the-gerson-therapy/

Robb Wolf - https://robbwolf.com/

United Kingdom bulk herb supplier - https://www.organicherbtrading.com/

United States herb supplier - https://mountainroseherbs.com/catalog/herbs-spices/bulk

Find Raw Milk Supplier - https://www.realmilk.com/raw-milk-finder/

Hippocrates - https://www.britannica.com/biography/Hippocrates

Section 7

Index